KETO
DIET
SERIES

A beginners Guide To Ketogenic Diet Cookbook For A Rapid and Healthy Weight Loss Journey

By Sara Clark

Chapter 3: Dinner Recipes 55

Chapter 4: Snacks Recipes 77

Chapter 6: Salad Recipes 118

Chapter 7: Smoothies Recipes 139

Chapter 8: Breakfast Recipes 148

Chapter 9: Lunch Recipes 161

Chapter 10: Dinner Recipes 182

Chapter 11: Snacks Recipes 207

Chapter 12: Soup Recipes 229

Chapter 13: Salad Recipes 255

Chapter 14: Smoothies Recipes 275

Chapter 15: Breakfast Recipes 284

Chapter 18: Snacks Recipes...................... 345

Introduction

As modern problems need a modern solution, and the same approach is required to deal with modern health diseases like cancer, obesity, heart disease, and alike. The introduction of new technology has provided immense ease to humanity, reducing workforce application for carrying out laborious tasks. The introduction of new powerful, multi-purpose, and easy to use machines has replaced humans working in various workspace fields. There are certain classes of people for whom technology has proven to be more beneficial than they have imagined. Simultaneously, there is a wide extended class of people who have lost their job and are suffering from earning their livelihood.

Furthermore, there exists a class whose workload has been decreased while they are retaining their job. Workspace for the latter described class has mostly been restricted to a single chair from where they deal with their respective computers to perform their assigned tasks throughout their extensive working hours. Although their workload has been decreased compared to the past, they had to perform tasks using physical energy, which indirectly helped them remain physically fit while maintaining good health. Their job was a sort of exercise. However, they are at more because they are at ease physically, and their physical workload is taken upon by machines. This ease has not reduced their work hours, and they had to work for an extended time that does not allows them to make out some time for themselves to exercise regularly to maintain their physical and mental health. Nowadays, people are more prone to diseases, and due to changes in surroundings, new diseases are finding ground making people remain more conscious about their health. Obesity is one of the most commonly reported diseases nowadays. Patients complain of an increase in their weight, swelling of their belly, and misalignment of their body structure, making them look ugly and unconfident. Once this disease reaches its climax, it triggers several other diseases like heart disease, blood pressure variation, diabetes and many more. Technology has always helped human beings counter their problem, so in this case, there are certain methods to easily get rid of this disease. The Keto diet is one of the most appreciated techniques to increase weight problems with no side effects. Keto diet focuses on curbing the intake of carbohydrate and allowing a moderate level of protein while encouraging fat intake because food intake with this kind of nutrition will change the metabolic pathway of extracting energy from glucose breakdown to breakdown of stored fats which in turn will cause a reduction in weight of an individual. This diet includes a meal plan in which different dishes are proposed for a patient whose ingredients are measured according to the nutrients mentioned above. This will help the patient to burn their fat quickly without providing room for their replacement, hence triggering the weight loss without much hard work. This technique demands determination and discipline to follow the diet plan religiously; otherwise, patients may have to suffer its side effects.

KETO DIET
FOOD PYRAMID

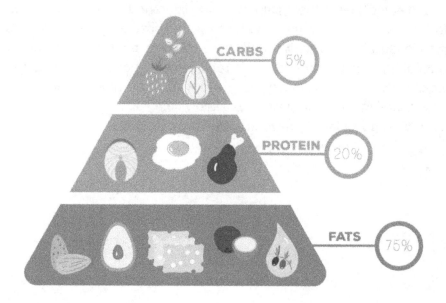

Chapter 1: Breakfast Recipes

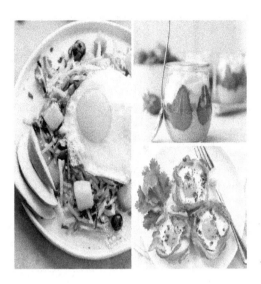

1. Breakfast Casserole

Ready in: 85 mins

Servings: 12

Difficulty: Difficult

INGREDIENTS

- 2 cup shredded ham

- Salt to taste

- Pepper to taste

- 1 tsp season salt

- 1 ½ cup grated jack cheese

- 12 eggs

- 24 oz chopped potatoes

- 1 ½ cup grated cheddar cheese

DIRECTIONS

1. Add pepper and salt in chopped and frozen potatoes and pour in a pan.

2. Take another bowl, whisk eggs in it and then add all the remaining ingredients.

3. Pour it over the frozen potatoes and refrigerate overnight.

4. Heat the oven at 350°C and bake it for 90 minutes.

5. Serve and enjoy it.

NUTRITION: Calories: 225 kcal Fat: 18 g Protein: 14 g Carbohydrates: 2 g

2. Onion Omelet

Ready in: 10 minutes

Servings: 2

Difficulty: Easy

INGREDIENTS

- White pepper to taste

- Three eggs

- 1 tsp soy sauce

- 1tpsp oyster sauce

- Sesame oil (sprinkle)

- 2tpsp cooking oil

- One diced onions

DIRECTIONS

1. Take a bowl to add pepper, salt, sesame oil, oyster, and soya sauce.

2. Add finely chopped onion and mix it.

3. Cook each side for 3 minutes.

4. Serve and enjoy.

NUTRITION: Calories: 240 cal Fat: 18.4 g Protein: 14 g Carbs: 4.6 g

3. Bacon and Eggs

Ready in: 20 minutes

Servings: 4

Difficulty: Easy

INGREDIENTS

- 150 g bacon

- Salt taste

- Pepper to taste

- Eight eggs

- ¼ cup parsley

- ½ cup tomatoes

DIRECTIONS

1. Take a pan and fry bacon over medium to low heat.

2. Cook eggs in a separate pan with a sunny side up, and then add tomatoes to it.

3. Add the seasoning you want and serve it hot.

NUTRITION: Calories: 370 kcal Fat: 31 g Protein: 20 g Carbs: 1 g

4. Eggs with Ham

Ready in: 20 minutes

Servings: 4

Difficulty: Easy

INGREDIENTS

- 1 cup cheese, shredded

- ¼ cup olive oil

- One minced jalapeno pepper

- Eight beaten eggs

- Pepper to taste

- Salt to taste

- 3tbsp milk

- ½ cup finely chopped ham

- ¼ cup salt

DIRECTIONS

1. Take a bowl and beat eggs, black pepper, seasoned salt, and salt in it.

2. Sauté jalapeno in olive oil over medium flame for 3 to 4 mins.

3. Then add ham to it and cook for 2 mins.

4. Pour the mixture of egg in jalapeno mixture and cook for 4 to 5 mins.

5. Sprinkle half cheese over it and cook till cheese melts.

6. Turn off the flame and add the remaining amount of cheese over it.

7. Serve and enjoy.

NUTRITION: Calories: 400 cal Fat: 33 g Protein: 23 g Carbs: 1.8 g

5. Chia Oatmeal

Prep time: 5 minutes

Chill time: 8 hours

Servings: 1

Difficulty: Difficult

INGREDIENTS

- One sliced banana

- ¼ tsp vanilla

- ¾ cup almond milk, unsweetened

- 2tbsp almonds, sliced and toasted

- 1/3 cup oats

- 2 tsp honey

- 2tbsp cranberries, dried

- 1tbsp chia seeds

DIRECTIONS

1. Combine all the ingredients in a mixing bowl.

2. Stir the mixture thoroughly and refrigerate it overnight.

3. Garnish with almonds and banana before serving.

NUTRITION: Calories: 485 cal Fat: 15 g Protein: 10 g Carbs: 85 g

6. Curry Cauliflower Rice Bowls

Ready in: 15 mins

Servings: 4

Difficulty: Easy

INGREDIENTS

- ½ cup green peas

- 3tbsp olive oil

- 12 oz. cauliflower rice

- ½ cup chopped bell pepper (red)

- ¼ tablespoon ground coriander

- ½ cup chopped onion

- Salt to taste

- ½ cup chopped onion, Sweet

- 1 ½ tablespoon curry powder

- Two crushed garlic cloves

- ¼tbsp turmeric powder

DIRECTIONS

1. Sauté onion and bell pepper in a pan for 5-6 mins in olive oil.

2. Then add garlic powder in it and sauté it for 2 mins.

3. Take a bowl and mix salt, curry powder, coriander, and turmeric.

4. Add peas, seasoning mix, and cauliflower rice in the pan and cook it for 7-8 mins over medium flame.

5. Serve and enjoy.

NUTRITION: Calories: 101 kcal Fat: 7.5 g Protein: 2.9 g Carbs: 5 g

7. Pesto Scrambled Eggs

Ready in: 10 minutes

Servings: 1

Difficulty: Easy

INGREDIENTS

- ½ tsp pesto

- 1tbsp oil

- Salt as required

- Pepper as required

- One beaten egg

- ½ cup cheese, shredded

DIRECTIONS

1. Combine all the ingredients in a bowl.

2. Pour this mixture into the pan and cook it for 5-6 mins over medium flame with continuous stirring.

3. Turn off the flame and stir it in pesto.

NUTRITION: Calories: 319 cal Fat: 29.1 g Protein: 13.8 g Carbs: 0.9 g

8. Egg and Mushroom Breakfast

Ready in: 10 mins

Servings: 3

Difficulty: Easy

INGREDIENTS

- ½ cup onion, chopped

- Two eggs

- Pepper as required

- Salt as required

- 2tbsp olive oil

- Parsley

DIRECTIONS

1. Sauté onions in a pan over medium flame.

2. Then add mushrooms in it and cook for 5-6 mins.

3. Take a bowl, beat eggs in it and then add black pepper and salt it.

4. Pour this mixture into the pan and cook for 5-8 mins.

5. When eggs are cooked, remove heat and serve it.

NUTRITION: Calories: 186.9 cal Fat: 14.3 g Protein: 12 g Carbs: 12 g

9. Cheesy Sausage Potatoes

Ready in: 20 minutes

Servings: 8

Difficulty: Easy

INGREDIENTS

- 2 cups cheese

- One chopped onion

- 3 lb. potatoes, sliced

- ¼ cup butter

- 1 lb. pork sausage

DIRECTIONS

1. Boil potatoes in a pan, then reduce the flame and simmer them for 7-8 mins.

2. Take another pan, add onion and crumbled sausage. Cook till meat is fully cooked.

3. Now add sausage mixture and potatoes in a baking dish and top with cheese.

4. Bake this mixture at 350° for 8 mins.

NUTRITION: Calories: 252 cal Fat: 13 g Protein: 9 g Carbs: 26 g

10. Almond and Strawberry Oatmeal

Ready in: 8 minutes

Servings: 1

Difficulty: Easy

INGREDIENTS

- Strawberries

- 1 cup water or milk

- ¼ tsp vanilla extract

- ½ cup oats

- Salt to taste

- Few almonds

- ½ banana

- ½ tsp almond extract

DIRECTIONS

1. Boil milk in a pan and add oats to it over medium flame.

2. Add mashed banana to the pan.

3. After few minutes, add salt, vanilla, and almond extract and stir it.

4. Now add sliced strawberries into oatmeal.

5. Keep on heating till the desired consistency is obtained.

6. Add desired toppings and serve them.

NUTRITION: Calories: 282 cal Fat: 12.4 g Protein: 5.6 g Carbs: 33.9 g

Chapter 2: Lunch Recipes

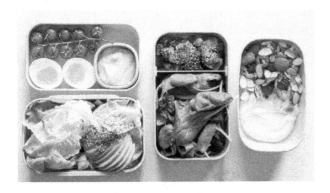

1. Curry Pork and Kale

Ready in: 25 minutes

Servings: 5

Difficulty: Easy

INGREDIENTS

- One onion

- One packet of brown lentils

- 240 g pork

- One packet tomato

- One container pasanda seasoning

- 200 ml coconut milk

- One packet ginger

- One green onion

- One packet chicken broth crumb

- 2 Naan

- 100 g kale

DIRECTIONS

1. Preheat your 400 Fahrenheit oven. Heat a drizzle of oil over med to high heat in a frying pan.

2. Add the ground pork when hot and season with salt and pepper. Cook for 4-5 mins, until golden brown. To break it up as it cooks, use a wooden spoon.

3. Halve the peel and slice the onion thinly when the pork is browning.

4. The garlic is peeled and rubbed

5. Drain and rinse these lentils in a sieve.

6. Stir in the onion until the pork is browned. Cook until softened, 4-5 mins with the pork mince. Stir in the garlic, pasanda pepper, tomato puree, and ginger puree. Mix and cook for 1 min, then add coconut milk, water, and powdered chicken stock. Stir in the lentils, bring to a boil and simmer until slightly reduced 3-4 mins.

7. Meanwhile, cut and thinly slice the spring onion.

8. Into the pork mixture, mix the kale.

9. Cover with a cap or some tin foil and cook for 3-4 mins until the kale is tender. Meanwhile, to heat up, pop the naan into your oven for 3-4 mins.

10. Taste the curry and season with salt and pepper.

NUTRITION: Calories: 874 kcal Fat: 39.0 g Protein: 42 g Carbs: 85 g

2. Mustard and Rosemary Pork Chops with Swiss Chard

Ready in: 30 minutes

Servings: 4

Difficulty: Easy

INGREDIENTS

- 2 tbsp mustard

- Four pork lions, cubes

- 1 tbsp butter

- 3 tbsp breadcrumbs

- 1 tbsp rosemary

- Two dried garlic

- 1/2 cup onion, chopped.

- 1 tbsp honey

- 1 Swiss cluster chard

- 1 tsp lemon

- 2 tsp wine vinegar

DIRECTIONS

1. Preheat the oven and place a rack in the top third of the oven to broil. Powder the pork with half of the salt and pepper on both sides. In a large oven-safe skillet, heat half of the butter over a med pan and cook the pork until golden, 3 to 4 mins. Remove from the heat, brush tops with mustard, then scatter uniformly overtop with rosemary and breadcrumbs. Place the skillet beneath the broiler till the pork is fried and golden, around 2 mins.

2. Meanwhile, over moderate melt, heat the remaining butter in a broad deep-sided frying pan. Add the onion, garlic, and chard stem and simmer for 2 to 3 mins, until tender.

3. Stir in the chard leaves and 30 mL of water. Season with salt and pepper to taste, cover and simmer until tender, about 5 mins.

NUTRITION: Calories: 230 kcal Fat: 7 g Protein: 27 g Carbs: 14 g

3. Pork Fried Cauliflower Rice

Ready in: 25 minutes

Servings: 5

Difficulty: Easy

INGREDIENTS

- Salt to taste

- 2 tsp sesame oil

- 1 lb pork

- 2 cups cabbage

- Pepper to taste

- Four sliced onion

- One sliced carrot

- 2 tsp sliced ginger

- Four bulbs of garlic, sliced

- 2 tbsp soy sauce

- 4 cups cauliflower rice

DIRECTIONS

1. In a med saucepan, heat the sesame seed. Add pork and cook until heated through and no longer green, breaking it up as it heats. It's going to take 6-8 mins.

2. Cabbage, onions, green onion, garlic, and ginger are added. Once the cabbage and carrots are tender, simmer for 4-5 mins.

3. Stir in the rice from the cauliflower and press it into the pan. Let it cook without changing it for 3-4 mins before the rice starts to brown. Mix and repeat then.

4. Stir in the sauce with the soy. As required, taste and add more soy sauce.

NUTRITION: Calories: 286 kcal Fat: 12 g Protein: 27 g Carbs: 13 g

4. Asian Pork Meatballs with Noodles and Vegetable Rice

Ready in: 30 minutes

Servings: 2

Difficulty: Easy

INGREDIENTS

- One slice ginger

- Three onion

- One lime

- One bulbs garlic

- 1 cluster coriander

- One carrot

- ½ package Rice Noodle

- One bunch coriander

- 3 tbsp soy sauce

- 250 g pork mince

- One packet Mangetout

- 15 g Breadcrumbs

- 25 g peanuts

- 2 tbsp soy sauce

DIRECTIONS

1. Thinly slice the root and cut it from the spring onion. Peel the ginger and garlic and finely grind them. Zest and cut the lime in two. Remove the carrot ends and grate coarsely. Chop the coriander loosely. Make the kettle boil.

2. Placed them in a bowl with the rice noodles. To fully submerge them, spill sufficiently hot water over the noodles, then cover them with cling film or a pan. Leave to the side before depleting in a colander for 8-10 mins

3. In a mixing cup, pop the pork mince and add half of the garlic, half of the spring onion, half of the ginger, and all of the lime zest. Add a fourth of the amount of soy to all the panko breadcrumbs and mix well to combine. Shape the mixture into four meatballs for every person.

4. Heat a drizzle of oil over med to high heat in a large cooking pot. Add the meatballs and fry, rotating periodically, 8-10 mins, until browned all over. Add the remaining spring onion, ginger, and garlic along with the mange tout and carrot until the meatballs are golden brown, then stir-fry all for 1 min.

5. Add the ketchup and leftover soy sauce, mix and boil for 2-3 mins, then tip in the noodles and half the coriander. Squeeze half of the lime into the juice. Toss until the noodles are piping hot to mix and heat,2-3 mins.

6. Serve it in sprinkle and bowls over the rest of the coriander and the peanuts. With a slice of the remaining lime, serve.

NUTRITION: Calories: 686 kcal Fat: 27.0 g Protein: 36 g Carbs: 76 g

5. Jalapeno-Garlic-Onion Cheeseburgers

Ready in: 25 minutes

Servings: 4

Difficulty: Easy

INGREDIENTS

- ½ cup sliced jalapeno

- 2 tbsp garlic

- One chopped onion

- 1 lb beef

- 1 cup jack cheese

- Four hamburger buns

DIRECTIONS

1. Heat the grill pan over high heat.

2. Take a bowl and mix pepper, onion, ground beef, and garlic in it. Make small patties from it.

3. Grill the patties for 3-5 minutes and top with cheese.

4. Serve with buns.

5. Enjoy.

NUTRITION: Calories: 474 Cal Fat: 26.8 g Protein: 31.6 g Carbs: 24.8 g

6. Jalapeno Popper Chicken

Ready in: 35 minutes

Servings: 6

Difficulty: Easy

INGREDIENTS

- 1.5 lb chicken boneless

- salt & pepper

- 8 oz cream cheese

- 2 tbsps milk

- 1/2 tsp garlic powder

- ½ cup chopped jalapeno peppers

- 1/2 cup of cooked bacon

- 1 cup of cheddar

DIRECTIONS

1. Take the baking dish & spray it with oil.

2. Put the chicken in layers over the baking dish and season with salt & pepper.

3. Take a bowl and mix garlic powder, cheese, and cream at room temperature.

4. Spread the mixture on chicken and sprinkle cheese, peppers, and bacon over it.

5. Cover the dish with aluminum foil and bake for 35-40 minutes.

6. Serve and enjoy.

NUTRITION: Calories: 349 Cal Fat: 26 g Protein: 28 g Carbs: 1 g

7. Perfect Sirloin Beef Roast

Ready in: 1 hour 45 minutes

Servings: 12

Difficulty: Difficult

INGREDIENTS

- 7 lb beef sirloin roast

- One onion

- Two celery ribs

- Two carrots

- 3 tbsp garlic

- 1/2 cup of water

Spice mix

- 3 tbsp onion flakes

- 2 tbsp oregano

- 1 tbsp peppercorns

- 1 tbsp coriander

- 1 tbsp Himalayan salt

- 1½ tsp chili pepper flakes

DIRECTIONS

1. Grind the spices & mix.

2. Clean the meat and spread spices over it. Cover the meat with plastic and put it in the fridge for one whole day.

3. Take a baking dish and put onion, carrot, garlic and celery, and some water in it. Place the meat over it.

4. Bake it in preheated oven for 10-15 minutes.

6. Put aluminum foil and roast in the oven for more than 30 minutes.

7. Take out the dish from the oven and place it over the cutting board.

8. Remove the carve.

9. Serve and enjoy.

NUTRITION: Calories: 312 Cal Fat: 8 g Protein: 53 g Carbs: 3 g

8. Country Fried Steak

Ready in: 20 minutes

Servings: 6

Difficulty: Easy

INGREDIENTS

- One 1/2lbs steak

- 1 cup of all-purpose flour

- 1 tsp paprika

- 1 1/2 tsp salt

- 1 1/4 tsp pepper

- Butter

- 2 1/2 cups milk

- Three eggs

- 4 tbsp oil

DIRECTIONS

1.   Take 3-4 bowls and put eggs and half a cup of milk with one flour cup.

2.   Mix one tbsp of salt and pepper along with paprika in the flour mixture.

3. Dip the steaks in milk first and then in the flour mixture.

4. Now dip the steaks in eggs and again into the flour.

5. Take a large skillet and heat a small amount of olive oil over medium flame.

6. Fry the steaks in the skillet for 10-15 minutes till they get brown color.

7. Melt the butter with a small amount of oil in the pan.

8. Add milk and stir continuously till it gets a boil and becomes thick.

9. Remove it from the stove.

10. Serve the steaks with gravy and mashed potatoes.

11. Enjoy.

NUTRITION: Calories: 272.2 Cal Fat: 139 g Protein: 9.1 g Carbs: 24.2 g

9. Asian Pork Meatballs

Ready in: 60 minutes

Servings: 5

Difficulty: Medium

INGREDIENTS

- 3 tbsp fish sauce

- 2 tbsp honey

- One bulb chopped garlic

- Four crushed onion

- 1 tsp cornflour

- 2 tsp crushed lemongrass

- 2 tbsp crushed coriander

- 1 tbsp crushed mint

- For sauce

- 1 tsp crushed coriander

- 2 tbsp lemon juice

- Three chopped onion

- 1 tsp sesame oil

- 2 tbsp soy sauce

DIRECTIONS

1. Make meatballs. In a non-stick frying pan, melt the honey softly, add the fish sauce and stir to make a syrup.

2. In a bowl, put the pork and add in the honey syrup, green onions, garlic, lemongrass, cornflower, mint, and cilantro. Add salt and black pepper to the blend and season.

3. Make it 20 balls and place them on a paper-lined tray, 30 mins to relax. All the ingredients are combined to make the sauce and put aside.

4. Brush the olive oil on the balls and fry each side for 3-4 mins. Serve.

NUTRITION: Calories: 51 kcal Fat: 3 g Protein: 5 g Carbs: 3 g

10. Eggplant and Chili Garlic Port Stir Fry

Ready in: 30 minutes

Servings: 4

Difficulty: Easy

INGREDIENTS

- 1 lb eggplant

- 3 tbsp olive oil

- Three bulbs garlic

- ½ chopped onion,

- One zucchini

- ½ lb pork

- 2 tbsp fish sauce

- 2 tbsp garlic sauce

- Black pepper to taste

- 1 tbsp rice vinegar

DIRECTIONS

1. Over med-high heat, heat a skillet. Add two tsp of olive oil, then add the eggplant to the mixture. Cook for 3-5 min until the eggplant is seared, rotating periodically. Take the eggplant outside the pan and move it aside.

2. Then add the remaining olive oil to the skillet, and stir in the garlic and onions. Heat until soft, and then stir in the ground pork for 1 min or until soft. Cook until the pork is browned, or around 3 min.

3. Mix in the zucchini, sauce with chili garlic, sauce with fish, and vinegar with rice. Cook till the zucchini is soft, about 3 mins. Mix in the eggplant and continue to cook for 2 mins or until some of the eggplant sauce has been drained by heating and frying.

NUTRITION: Calories: 452 kcal Fat: 23 g Protein: 29.8 g Carbs: 33.3 g

11. Thai Shrimp and Eggplant Stir Fry

Ready in: 34 minutes

Servings: 4

Difficulty: Medium

INGREDIENTS

- 1 ½ tbsp fish sauce

- 2 tbsp lemon juice

- 5 tsp peanut oil

- 1 ½ tsp sugar

- Three eggplants

- 1 lb shrimp

- Two chilies

- Five bulbs garlic

- 1 cup basil leaves

- One sliced spring onion

- Rice noodles, cooked.

- Slice of lime wedges

DIRECTIONS

1. Whisk the fish sauce, sugar, lime juice, and water in a small dish.

2. Heat 1 tbsp oil on med heat until quite hot in a 12-inches non-stick skillet; swirl to cover the skillet. Add shrimp and stir-fry for about 3 mins.

3. Into the skillet and half of the eggplant, add oil. Cook for an additional min, uninterrupted, then stir-fry for 30 secs. Move it to a shrimp dish. Add two additional tsp. Of oil; repeat for remaining eggplant. In the middle, make a well and add the remaining oil, garlic, chili, and scallion—Stir-fry for around 1 min.

4. To the skillet, add the lobster, eggplant, and sauce. Cook, toss well until fully heated 30 sec-1 min. Serve with rice noodles and lime wedges.

NUTRITION: Calories: 209 kcal Fat: 10 g Protein: 18 g Carbs: 12 g

12. Lemon Chicken with Artichokes and Kale

Ready in: 25 minutes

Servings: 1

Difficulty: Easy

INGREDIENTS

- 3 tbsp olive oil

- 6 oz kale

- ½ tsp black pepper

- 5 oz chicken

- 9 oz artichokes

- ¼ tsp salt

- 1 tbsp decide thyme,

- One lemon

- ¼ tsp red pepper powder

- 2 oz cheese

DIRECTIONS

1. With the oven rack in the top spot, preheat the broiler to high. In the oven, put a rimmed baking dish.

2. In a cup, combine the kale and 1 tbsp oil; rub the leaves until slightly wilted with your fingertips.

3. Sprinkle black salt and pepper with the chicken. Take the pan from the oven very carefully. To the plate, add 1 tbsp of oil; turn the pan to coat. Add the chicken to the saucepan; boil for five mins.

4. Add the artichokes and pieces of lemon to the pan. Sprinkle oil and thyme. Broil before you're done with chicken, 10 to 12 mins. Place the chicken on a cutting panel. Add the kale mixture to the pan; broil for 3 to 5 mins until the kale is fried and the sides are crisp.

5. Send the chicken back to the pan; add cheese, lemon juice, thyme, and pepper.

NUTRITION: Calories: 417 kcal Fat: 19 g Protein: 40 g Carbs: 20 g

13. Crispy Roast Duck with Fennel and Orange

Ready in: 75 minutes

Servings: 5

Difficulty: difficult

INGREDIENTS

- One orange

- 1 Duck

- One bottle cider

- One fennel, slice into 8th pieces

- ¼ cup chopped apricots

- 1 cup chicken soup

- 2 tbsp sugar

- Four spring thyme

- Olive oil

- Salt to taste

DIRECTIONS

1. To 400 Fahrenheit, pre-heat the oven.

2. Set the duck down on the other side of the skin of an oven tray. Place the orange with some sea salt inside the duck cavity. Place the mixture in the oven and prepare it for 30 mins. Switch to the side of the skin after 30 mins and cook for another hour.

3. Place all the remaining ingredients in the pan and bake for 45 minutes.

4. If the fennel has been braised, cut it, keep it warm and pass the liquid to a saucepan. Add the starch, bring it to a boil, and simmer. Reduce to a clotted sauce and to serve, set aside.

5. Carve the breast and the legs out of the duck to serve. Cut the breasts and place them next to the braised fennel on a platter.

NUTRITION: Calories: 514 kcal Fat: 43 g Protein: 15 g Carbs: 18 g

14. Duck Chili

Ready in: 80 minutes

Servings: 6

Difficulty: difficult

INGREDIENTS

- 3 tbsp duck Fat

- 1 Duck Breast

- 1/8 cup chopped chili

- One crushed onion

- 1 tbsp chopped garlic

- 1 tbsp cumin

- Three chopped carrots

- ½ tbsp oregano

- 1 tbsp paprika

- 1 cup beef broth

- 8 oz tomato juice

- 9 oz kidney beans

- 1 tbsp vinegar

- 1 cup crushed mushrooms

- One crushed green pepper

DIRECTIONS

1. Grind the duck breast by hand. Put for 5 mins in the fridge. Remove the substance and grind it with a small knife. Break the duck breast into thin slices across the width and then again across the thickness. Chopping until you have a clean, coarse grind is the final stage.

2. In a deep dutch oven, melt the duck fat over med-low heat and add the onion—Cook for 10 mins, or till your potatoes are tender. Alternatively, you might make this duck chili dish in a crockpot or slow cooker.

3. Cook for 5 mins after adding the garlic and carrots.

4. Flakes of red pepper, cumin, paprika, chili powder, and oregano are added. Then, prepare 3 mins of duck chili. Next, add broth, tomato sauce, and vinegar. Stir, then cook for 40 mins and cover.

5. Mushrooms and bell peppers are added. Let the duck chili boil for 15 more mins. Immediately serve.

NUTRITION: Calories: 340 kcal Fat: 8 g Protein: 19 g Carbs: 51 g

Chapter 3: Dinner Recipes

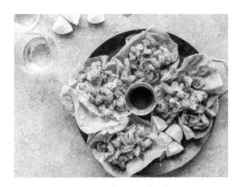

1. Beer and Mushroom Instant Pot Roast

Ready in: 140 minutes

Servings: 6

Difficulty: Difficult

INGREDIENTS

- 3 cups onion soup

- 4 lb Blade Roast

- One sliced onion

- 2 tbsp olive oil

- 2 Stalks celery

- 1 tsp sauce

- 1 tbsp garlic paste

- 10.75 oz mushroom soup

- 2 cup bottle wine

- 10 oz mushroom

DIRECTIONS

1. Here for this recipe, the instant pot is used. Olive oil is added to it and turns it on. After burning roast in it, turn off the instant pot.

2. Then all available vegetables are added.

3. Different ingredients like beer, Worcestershire sauce, and soup are mixed in a measuring cup.

4. Then this mixture is poured on the roast.

5. For almost two hours, cook the roast by turning on the instant pot's meat button while keeping in view that pressure should be high.

6. Release steam produced in the pot it could be done manually or naturally as well.

7. Then take a saucepan and add pour sauce in it (about 2-3 cups). Boil it for u5 to 6 minutes.

8. And then, take one teaspoon of cornstarch to add it to a quarter cup of water. Pour it on the boiling sauce and cook it for a time.

9. Roast beef is ready and serves to guests along with tasty gravy.

NUTRITION: Calories: 324 kcal Fat: 21 g Protein: 29 g Carbs: 2 g

2. Coconut Pork Curry

Ready in: 4 hours 40 minutes

Servings: 8

Difficulty: Difficult

INGREDIENTS

- 3 cups chicken soup

- 2 tbsp oil

- One sliced of onion

- 4 lb boneless pork

- Salt to taste

- 1 tbsp Grained curry powder

- Black pepper to taste

- 1 cup coconut milk

- Three cloves chopped Garlic

- 14 oz chopped tomatoes

- 3 tbsp chopped ginger

- ½ tsp turmeric powder

- Boil rice

DIRECTIONS

1. First of all, olive oil is heated in a skillet. Pork is flavored by mixing with table salt pepper. Divide the pork into two halves, add one of them in the skillet and cook it for about 12-15 minutes at moderate heat. Then similarly transfer the other half and brown it.

2. Then add 2 tbsp of fat to this browned pork skillet. Add certain other ingredients like garlic, curry, onion, cumin, and turmeric, and cook it at low heat. Continue stirring while cooking until you feel their fragrance. Separate all this mixture into a slow cooker. To make it tastier, add coconut milk, tomatoes, and tomato juice and then cook it in a small cooker for about 4 hours. Remove fat from the surface of stew. Your recipe is ready to serve it elegantly to your guests.

NUTRITION: Calories: 491 kcal Fat: 25 g Protein: 46 g Carbs: 21 g

3. Buffalo Pulled Pork with Bacon

Ready in: 4 Hours 10 minutes

Servings: 10

Difficulty: Difficult

INGREDIENTS

- 600g of bacon

- 2 lb pork shoulder

- ½ cup soy sauce

- ¾ cup hot sauce

- ½ cup ranch

DIRECTIONS

1. Bacon is first cooked and then make their small chops.

2. Add some ingredients like franks, sauce, and ranch dressing in a crockpot. Whisk them together, so they mix very well.

3. Then pour this mixture into a bacon crumble and put the pork into the crockpot.

4. Then allow it to heat at high pressure for four hours or at low up to 8 hours. on high for 4 hours or low 8 hours.

5. Freeze the pork and then serve it on bread sometimes; Pizza is also used.

NUTRITION: Calories: 91 kcal Fat: 7 g Protein: 3 g Carbs: 5 g

4. Pulled Pork Ofelia

Ready in: 6 hours 15 minutes

Servings: 5

Difficulty: Difficult

INGREDIENTS

-   3 lb pork shoulder

-   8 oz chopped onion

-   ¾ cup wine

-   1 tbsp garlic paste

-   ½ cup olive oil

- 2 tsp chopped thyme

- 2 tbsp coriander powder

- Black pepper to taste

- Salt to taste

- 2 tsp cinnamon

DIRECTIONS

1. Firstly, peel onions and make their small slices. Make tiny halves of garlic cloves. Mix these elements and soak them in the marinade. Take a freezer bag and add half of the onions to it.

2. Wash out the pork collar, make dry it, and shine it r with salt. Then put the pork collar in a freezer bag and soak it with marinade. Ensure there's no air in the bag and close it and position it in a mixing bowl. Then place the bowl in the refrigerator for 12 hours.

3. Turn on the oven and set its temperature at 125°C.

4. Then in an oven-specific dish, add meat onion mixture and marinade. Put this dish and heat it for 5-6hours. In a low cooker, meat is cooked in about 6-8 hours, and cooked meat will be very delectable.

5. It can be served with gravy.

NUTRITION: Calories: 758 kcal Fat: 59 g Protein: 40 g Carbs: 7 g

5. Stuffed Cabbage Rolls

Ready in: 80 minutes

Servings: 12

Difficulty: Difficult

INGREDIENTS

- ¼ cup water

- 1 lb ground beef

- One egg

- 1 tbsp onion powder

- 2 cups half cooked rice

- 26 oz Spaghetti sauce

- 1 tbsp garlic powder

- 1 cup Cabbage

- 1 tbsp black pepper

- 1 tbsp salt

DIRECTIONS

1. Take cabbage leaves, boil them for up to 4 mins, and put them in the cold water.

2. In a mixing bowl, add seasoning, ground beef, eggs, rice, and spaghetti, mix them all.

3. Place the ground beef mixture over the cabbage leaves one by the roll, then gently seal it with a toothpick.

4. In another pot, put spaghetti sauce, place the cabbage leaves, make another layer of spaghetti sauce, and a quarter cup of water simmer it for 1 hour at low flame.

5. Serve and enjoy it.

NUTRITION: Calories: 159.2 kcal Fat: 5 g Protein: 7 g Carbs: 25 g

6. Tofu and vegetable Satay Stir-fry

Ready in: 30 minutes

Servings: 5

Difficulty: Easy

INGREDIENTS

For the sauce

- One diced red chili

- 1 tbsp peanut butter

- Two diced garlic cloves

- One juiced lime

- Coriander leaves as required

- 2 tbsp ginger

- 1 tsp fish sauce

- 1 tbsp of soy sauce

- 1 tbsp yogurt

For stir-fry

- One diced leek

- 1 tsp coconut oil

- 2 cups noodles

- 400g firm tofu

- One diced pepper

- One diced carrot

- ½ diced of broccoli

DIRECTIONS

1. Put the ingredients of the sauce in a food processor and pulse it to make the sauce.

2. In a wok, add coconut oil and tofu and fry till it gets golden.

3. In another pan, boil the noodles according to packet details.

4. Now add vegetables in wok fry them but not lose the crunch of vegetables.

5. Add the sauce and stir it well. You may add water if required.

6. Add the noodles in wok and mix well.

NUTRITION: Calories: 97 kcal Fat: 7 g Protein: 1 g Carbs: 8 g

7. Spinach Russian Salad

Ready in: 40 minutes

Servings: 4

Difficulty: Medium

INGREDIENTS

- 4 tbsp olive oil

- Three tomatoes

- 200g block feta

- One minced garlic clove

- One diced green pepper

- Pitta bread to serve

- 1 tsp diced oregano

DIRECTIONS

1. Peel the tomatoes cut them into two pieces, scoop the seeds, now grate the seeds and the flash.

2. Season the tomatoes and do the scoping in a baking tray. Preheat the oven to 200 Fahrenheit.

3. Add cheese in garlicky tomatoes and cover them with tomato slices, oregano, salt, oil and chilies, and feta block. Bake it till it gets cooked.

NUTRITION: Calories: 243 kcal Fat: 21g Protein: 8 g Carbs: 4 g

8. Stovetop Spinach-Artichoke Dip

Ready in: 35 minutes

Servings: 5

Difficulty: Easy

INGREDIENTS

Bread bowl

- 1 Tbsp olive oil

- country loaf

- Salt to taste

Spinach-artichoke dip

- Black pepper to taste

- 1 tbsp unsalted butter

- 15 oz diced artichoke hearts

- One minced garlic clove

- 1 oz spinach

- 1 oz shredded cheese, parmesan

- Salt to taste

- Chips for serving

DIRECTIONS

1. Take the bread and make a hole in it to have a shape of bowl, now seasoned it with oil and salt and bake the bread for a half-hour

2. In a pan, add some butter and garlic fry. It nicely now adds artichokes spinach salt and stir it well.

3. In artichokes, add pepper parmesan and cream cheese till it gets melted.

4. Add the creamy sauce to the bread bowl, put some parmesan cheese over the top, and pepper bake it till it gets melted.

5. Enjoy the bread.

NUTRITION: Calories: 340 kcal Fat: 28 g Protein: 12 g Carbs: 10 g

9. Eggs in Purgatory

Ready in: 35 minutes

Servings: 4

Difficulty: Easy

INGREDIENTS

- 1/3 cup shredded cheese, parmesan

- 3 tbsp olive oil

- 2 tsp thyme, diced

- 1 ½ cups onion, diced

- ½ diced red pepper

- 9 oz artichoke hearts

- Salt to taste

- 28 oz smashed tomatoes

- Two smashed garlic clove

- 8 oz cubed potatoes

- Eight eggs

- 2 tbsp capers

DIRECTIONS

1. Take a large skillet with a good amount of oil, finely chopped onions, red pepper, add salt or taste, cook it for 10 mins.

2. Add diced tomatoes, chopped garlic, and artichokes in the pan and wait for simmer.

3. Add the boiled potatoes and capers in the skillet, mix it well with artichokes, season it with salt, and pepper sauce is ready.

4. In a glass baking dish, pour the artichokes sauce, make holes, and put the eggs in each of them.

5. Bake in the preheated oven around 350 Fahrenheit.

6. Enjoy the meal.

NUTRITION: Calories: 427 kcal Fat: 24.7 g Protein: 21.5 g Carbs: 5.7 g

10. Braised Artichokes with Tomatoes and Mint

Ready in: 30 minutes

Servings: 8

Difficulty: Easy

INGREDIENTS

- Two diced lemons

- 28 oz tomatoes

- ½ tsp chopped red pepper

- 1 ½ cups dry wine

- 2 tsp salt

- 12 anchovy fillets

- 1 cup olive oil

- Eight minced garlic cloves

- Six artichokes

- 1 cup mint leaves

DIRECTIONS

1. Take crushed tomatoes in a large pot, season them with red pepper flakes, wine, salt, water, and oil.

2. In a food processor, add artichokes and some cloves of garlic pulse it well. Now add coarse and half cup oil and pulse, make a perfect coarse pulse.

3. Take light green leaves of artichokes, trim the stem with a knife. Rub the trimmed area with lemon. Scoop the artichokes with the help of a spoon, and rub the inner part with lemon.

4. Make a layer of artichokes with past rubbing and merge in the crushed tomato mixture. Cook on medium flame, turn the artichokes from time to time.

5. Now put the chokes in the plater and cover it with foil. Turn the flame high till the sauce get thickens. Add the sauce over chokes and enjoy.

NUTRITION: Calories: 370 kcal Fat: 28 g Protein: 6 g Carbs: 19 g

11. Tandoori Lamb Meatloaf

Ready in: 75 minutes

Servings: 4

Difficulty: Difficult

INGREDIENTS

- 1 lb Lamb

- Five cloves chopped Garlic

- One chopped onion

- One chopped Serrano pepper

- 2 tsp red chili

- 5 tbsp tomato paste

- ¼ tsp cinnamon

- 1 tsp coriander powder

- Salt to taste

- 1 tsp turmeric powder

- Black pepper to taste

- Two eggs

- ¼ tsp cloves

- 1 tbsp sliced mint

- ½ tsp Nutmeg

Topping

- 1 tsp garlic powder

- 5 tbsp tomato paste

- Salt to taste

- ¼ cup water

- Black pepper to taste

DIRECTIONS

1. Whisk all elements together in a mixing bowl and disperse the mixture in the oiled loaf pan.

2. Roast loaf at 350 F for 60 minutes.

3. Take a saucepan and add ingredients to it to make ketchup.

4. When the loaf is cooked, put ketchup on it and then again place it in the oven for 10 minutes.

5. Remove it from the oven stand it for 5 minutes to let it be cool.

6. Take the loaf out of the pan and serve it.

NUTRITION: Calories: 360 kcal Fat: 21 g Protein: 26 g Carbs: 17 g

12. Grilled Lemon and Rosemary Lamb chops

Ready in: 4 hours 25 minutes

Servings: 8

Difficulty: Difficult

INGREDIENTS

- ¼ tsp cinnamon

- ½ cup yogurt

- 1 tbsp chili

- 1 tbsp lemon juice

- Four cloves chopped Garlic

- 1 tsp Oregano

- 2 tbsp chopped rosemary

- Salt to taste

- Eight lamb

- ½ tsp black pepper

DIRECTIONS

1. Take a mixing bowl and mix rosemary, black pepper, lemon juice, salt, garlic, cinnamon, lemon zest, lemon zest, and yogurt in it. Take a large freezer bag and add lamb chops rinsed with marinade; Seal the bag and make sure there's no air in it. Put this bag in the refrigerator and freeze it for 4 hours.

2. Ready the grill for baking and oil it.

3. Place lamb chops soaked in a marinade, rinsed with salt and black pepper on a preheated grill, and bake it until chops are browned.

4. Heat them for about 3-4 minutes.

NUTRITION: Calories: 198 kcal Fat: 13.6 g Protein: 15.3 g Carbs: 4.5 g

13. Grilled lamb in Paleo Mint Cream Sauce

Ready in: 25 minutes

Servings: 5

Difficulty: Easy

INGREDIENTS

- 1/8 cup coconut milk

- One rack lamb

- ¼ cup crushed mint

- 2 tbsp crushed Dill

- 1 tbsp lemon juice

- 2 tbsp red chili

DIRECTIONS

1. Take a mixing bowl and blend all these ingredients.

2. Place this mixture in a refrigerator.

3. Take a lamb rack and marinate it with oregano and olive oil.

4. Store it at room temperature before baking.

5. Make grill ready at an appropriate heat that will be enough to cook lamb chops.

6. Put lamb chops on a hot grill and heat them for approximately 4 minutes.

7. Use tongs to flip the lamb approximately; it takes 4 minutes for the side and 8 for others to cook properly.

8. Dip lamb chops in sauce and enjoy.

NUTRITION: Calories: 267 kcal Fat: 11.3 g Protein: 36 g Carbs: 2 g

14. Spinach Lamb and Cauliflower Curry

Ready in: 75 minutes

Servings: 4

Difficulty: Difficult

INGREDIENTS

- 1 tsp peanut oil

- Two cloves chopped Garlic

- One crushed onion

- ½ cup curry paste

- 425 g sliced Italian Tomatoes

- 700 g sliced lamb

- 125 g crushed Spinach

- 1 ½ cups water

- 145 g chicken peas

- 350 g cauliflower

- Salt to taste

- Crushed parsley

- Black pepper to taste

DIRECTIONS

1. Add the olive to a saucepan and heat it so that the pan is oil greased. Well, sliced onion and garlic are added and then stirred continuously for 1 minute until onions are softened. Then add a paste of curry, cook it, and stir until their fragrance comes out.

2. Then add lamb and bake it and make sure all sides are browned. Later on, add water and tomatoes and boil them. Keep the intensity of heat varying from low to medium and medium to high. Cook it for about 45 minutes with continuous stirring. And then add chickpeas and cauliflower in it and cook and stir for about 5 minutes. Also, add spinach and stir it.

3. Pour cooked spinach lamb and cauliflower curry in bowls and enjoy.

NUTRITION: Calories: 160 kcal Fat: 5.1 g Protein: 20.8 g Carbs: 7.8 g

15. Maple – Crusted Salmon Recipe

Ready in: 10minutes

Servings: 4

Difficulty: Easy

INGREDIENTS

- 1 tbsp red chili

- 2 tsp sugar

- 1 tbsp paprika

- Salt to taste

- 3 tbsp maple syrup

- 1 ½ lb salmon fillets

DIRECTIONS

1. First, turn on the oven and heat it at a specific temperature.

2. Ingredients for this recipe are chili powder, paprika, sugar, and salt

3. Take a mixing cup and blend all these ingredients and make their mixture.

4. Take salmon fillets and spray them liberally with a mixture of chili powder. Place your salmon onto a prepared baking sheet & broil for 6 to 9 mins, dependent on how thick the fillets are & how crispy you prefer the crust.

5. Then place salmon over the aluminum baking sheet and broil it up to 6-10 minutes. Time for broiling can vary depending on personal interest.

6. Take out salmon from the oven and remove maple syrup present on the top of the salmon. Place it again in the oven and broil for about 12 more minutes, so that maple syrup is bubbled out. Now, this Maple- the crusted salmon recipe is ready to serve.

NUTRITION: Calories: 300.21 kcal Fat: 11.29 g Protein: 34.27 g Carbs: 14.1 g

Chapter 4: Snacks Recipes

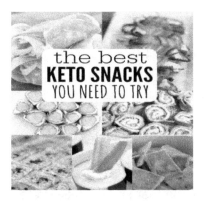

1. Baked mini–Bell Pepper

Ready in: 35 minutes

Servings: 5

Difficulty: Easy

INGREDIENTS

- 1 cup cheese

- 8 oz bell Pepper

- 1 tbsp chopped thyme

- 1 oz crushed chorizo

- 8 oz creamy cheese

- 2 tbsp olive oil

- ½ tbsp paprika paste

DIRECTIONS

1. Set your oven to 325 Fahrenheit.

2. Cut the bell peppers & remove all the core.

3. Combine the cream cheese, oil & spices in a container and mix in chorizo & herbs.

4. Place the mixture inside the empty bell pepper and sprinkle grated cheese.

5. Place the stuffed bell peppers in a baking tray sprayed with oil.

6. Bake in a preheated oven at 325 Fahrenheit for 18 minutes.

7. Serve and enjoy it.

NUTRITION: Calories: 411 kcal Fat: 38 g Protein: 12 g Carbs: 7 g

2. Caprese Snack

Ready in: 5 minutes

Servings: 5

Difficulty: Easy

INGREDIENTS

- Black pepper to taste

- 8 oz tomatoes

- 2 tbsp pesto

- 8 oz cheese

- Salt to taste

DIRECTIONS

1. Combine chopped tomatoes and diced cheese in a bowl.

2. Mix in pesto and toss well.

3. Sprinkle black pepper and salt to adjust the taste.

4. Serve and enjoy it.

NUTRITION: Calories: 218 kcal Fat: 16 g Protein: 14 g Carbs: 3 g

3. Caprese Bites

Ready in: 25 minutes

Servings: 5

Difficulty: Easy

INGREDIENTS

- Balsamic vinegar

- One sliced baguette

- Five chopped tomatoes

- 2 tbsp olive oil

- ½ cup crushed basil

- Salt to taste

- 12 oz chopped cheese

- Black pepper to taste

DIRECTIONS

1. Brush each bread slice with olive oil & put the slices in a baking tray.

2. Place the tray in a preheated oven set on the broiler and let it boil for four minutes.

3. Now add cheese slice and tomato slice followed by basil leaves and baguette slice over the broiled slice.

4. Drizzle with pepper and salt.

5. Bake in the preheated oven at 400 Fahrenheit for eight minutes.

6. Spread balsamic glaze and serve.

NUTRITION: Calories: 213 kcal Fat: 4 g Protein: 8 g Carbs: 36 g

4. Cauliflower Hash Brown

Ready in: 30 minutes

Servings: 12

Difficulty: Easy

INGREDIENTS

- ¼ tsp baking powder

- 1 lb cauliflower

- Two eggs

- 2 tbsp crushed onion

- ¼ tsp turmeric powder

- ½ cup cheddar, sliced

- ½ tsp garlic paste

- Salt to taste

- 3 tbsp coconut flour

DIRECTIONS

1. Grate the cauliflower in small pieces and add it to a bowl.

2. Now, place the bowl in the microwave for three minutes.

3. Spread the microwaved cauliflower over a paper towel for few minutes.

4. Remove the maximum moisture out of the cauliflower.

5. Add all the remaining ingredients in a bowl and cauliflower and mix well.

6. Make tiny balls from the mixture and place the balls in a baking tray lined with butter paper.

7. Bake in a preheated oven at 400 Fahrenheit for 15 minutes.

8. Serve and enjoy it.

NUTRITION: Calories: 45 kcal Fat: 2.4 g Protein: 3.1 g Carbs: 3.4 g

5. Sun-Dried Tomato Chicken Salad

Ready in: 25 minutes

Servings: 5

Difficulty: Easy

INGREDIENTS

- 1/3 cup of diced sun-dried tomatoes

- 2 cups of grated chicken, cooked

- 1/3 cup of mayonnaise

- 2 tbsp capers

- 2 tbsp parsley

- 2 tsp lemon juice

- Two onions, green

- ½ tsp black pepper

- ½ tsp salt

DIRECTIONS

1. In a medium mixing cup, combine all of the ingredients. To mix, stir all together. Season with salt and pepper to taste.

2. Store in an airtight jar for up to five days.

NUTRITION: Calories: 386.6 kcal Fat: 20.8 g Protein: 24.6 g Carbs: 20,1 g

6. Basic Crepes

Ready in: 30 minutes

Servings: 4

Difficulty: Easy

INGREDIENTS

- Two eggs

- 1 cup of all-purpose flour

- ½ cup of water

- ½ cup of milk

- 2 tbsp butter

- ¼ tsp salt

DIRECTIONS

1. Whisk the eggs & flour together in a wide mixing cup. Stir throughout the water or milk in a long, steady current. Combine the salt & butter in a mixing bowl and pound until smooth.

2. On medium to high flame heat frying pan or skillet. Using around 1/4 cup of batter per crepe, spill or shovel a batter on the griddle. Tilt the pan in some circular motion to uniformly brush the surface with batter.

3. Cook for around 2 mins, or until the bottom of the crepe is light brown. Turn, then cook another side after loosening with a spatula. Serve instantly.

NUTRITION: Calories: 216 kcal Fat: 9.2 g Protein: 7.4 g Carbs: 25. g

7. Whole-wheat Fettuccine with Kale and Goat's Cheese

Ready in: 45 minutes

Servings: 4.6

Difficulty: Medium

INGREDIENTS

- Salt to taste

- 2 tbsp olive oil

- Three diced onions, red

- 700 g lacinato kale, diced

- 340 g whole-wheat fettuccine

- Black pepper to taste

- 225 g goat cheese

Marinated Goat's Cheese

- 120 ml olive oil

- 225 g Goat's Cheese, diced

- ¼ tsp peppercorns

- Eight thyme sprigs

- Four bay leaves

- Three chopped garlic cloves

DIRECTIONS

1. Place the goat's cheese in the single-layer in a container to produce the goat's marinated cheese. Pour sufficient olive oil that fully coats the cheese along with garlic, thyme and bay leaf. Place it in the fridge until further use.

2. In such a wide frying pan on medium heat, melt the olive oil and add the pasta's onions. Cook for 10 minutes, or until the sides tend to brown. Add 1 tsp, reduce heat to medium-low, and simmer for another 15 to 20 minutes, or till onions are caramelized and soft. Meanwhile, put some big pot of the water to a boil, then season generously with salt. According to the box directions, when the onions have caramelized, add the fettuccine to the boiling water & cook for 10-12 mins, or until al dente. Send the pasta to the pan after draining.

3. While the pasta is cooking, stir the kale into the onions, cover, then cook for 6-8 minutes, or until the kale is soft, stirring once maybe twice. Toss the pasta with the onion and kale combination, three-quarters of a marinated goat's cheese, and plenty of black pepper. Season to taste with a tbsp or more of the cheese's oil marinade. Serve warm with the crumble of leftover goat's cheese on top of each mug.

NUTRITION: Calories: 323 kcal Fat: 26.6 g Protein: 5.5 g Carbs: 16.5 g

8. Vegetarian Gumbo

Ready in: 60 minutes

Servings: 9

Difficulty: Medium

INGREDIENTS

- Two sliced red bell pepper

- ½ cup of butter

- 2/3 cup of all-purpose flour

- One chopped onion, white

- Two sliced celery stalks

- Five smashed garlic cloves

- 1 cup of okra, diced

- One diced cauliflower

- 3 cups of vegetable broth

- 14 oz tomatoes, toasted

- 1 lb. chopped mushrooms

- ½ tsp thyme, dried

- 2 tsp Cajun seasoning

- One bay leaf

- ½ tsp cayenne

- Pepper

- Salt

DIRECTIONS

1. Melt the butter over med to high heat in a bowl. In a different bowl, whisk together the flour & salt until well mixed. Cook for another 20 minutes, stirring continuously, or when the roux mixture achieves a rich amber-brown hue. Keep a careful watch on roux at all stages and should the fire if it appears to be cooked too fast or tends to smell burnt.

2. As soon as the roux is prepared, stir throughout the okra, bell peppers, onion, celery, & garlic until it is well mixed. Cook, stirring after 10 to 15 seconds, for another 5 minutes, or till these vegetables have softened.

3. Progressively whisk into vegetable stock till the broth is creamy. The cayenne, thyme, cauliflower, seasoning, onions, mushrooms, & bay leaf are then included. Stir until it is well mixed, then boil till the soup hits a simmer.

4. Decrease the heat to almost medium to low and proceed to cook the gumbo for another 5-10 mins, or till these vegetables are soft. If required, season with additional salt, pepper, or/and cayenne.

5. Serve directly over barley, served with a sprinkling of green onions. Please put it in the fridge for three days or freeze for three months until switching to a locked jar.

NUTRITION: Calories: 494 kcal Fat: 24.2 g Protein: 16.3 g Carbs: 56 g

9. Potatoes Pancakes

Ready in: 20 minutes

Servings: 6

Difficulty: Easy

INGREDIENTS

- One egg

- Four potatoes

- One onion, yellow

- 2 tbsp all-purpose flour

- 1 tsp salt

- 2 cups of vegetable oil

- Black pepper

DIRECTIONS

1. In a broad mixing dish, finely grind the potatoes and onion. Every extra liquid should be extracted.

2. Combine the salt, egg, & black pepper in a mixing dish. Apply sufficient flour to thicken the paste, around 2-4 tbsp overall.

3. Preheat the oven to a low temperature of around 200 Fahrenheit.

4. Throughout the bottom of the heavy skillet, melt one-fourth-inch inch oil on medium to high heat. Through the hot oil, drop two to three one-fourth cup mounds and flatten and fry.

NUTRITION: Calories: 283 kcal Fat: 8.4 g Protein: 6.5 g Carbs: 46.7 g

10. Eggplant Gratin

Ready in: 60 minutes

Servings: 5

Difficulty: Medium

INGREDIENTS

- 13 cup bread crumbled

- Three diced eggplants

- 1 tsp Lemon Juice

- Four chopped tomatoes

- 1 tsp crushed thyme

- ¼ cup olive oil

- One bulb chopped garlic

- Salt to taste

- 4 oz cheese

- Black pepper to taste

DIRECTIONS

1. Combine tomatoes, salt, thyme, eggplant, olive oil, zest, pepper, and garlic in a bowl. Mix well.

2. To a baking tray, transfer the mixture & sprinkle goat cheese, panko, and olive oil over them.

3. In a preheated oven, bake it at 400 Fahrenheit for 55 minutes.

4. Serve and enjoy it.

NUTRITION: Calories: 302 kcal Fat: 24.3 g Protein: 9.4 g Carbs: 14 g

11. Cheesy Eggplant

Ready in: 45 minutes

Servings: 2

Difficulty: Medium

INGREDIENTS

- ½ cup tomato sauce
- Olive oil
- ¼ cup cheese
- ¾ lb Chopped eggplant
- Black pepper to taste
- One egg
- ½ cups chopped parmesan
- ¼ cup heavy cream
- Salt to taste

DIRECTIONS

1. At first, preheat your oven to 400 Fahrenheit.

2. Heat almost 1/8-inches of the olive oil in a large frying pan on med heat. When the oil is about smoking, you can add some slices of the eggplant & cook, turn once, till they're finely browned on sides & cooked thoroughly, about 5 mins. But be careful. It sometimes splatters. Shift those cooked slices of eggplant to thick tissue paper to drain it. Add some more oil, then heat & add some more eggplants till all of the slices have been cooked.

3. Meanwhile, in a small bowl, mix ricotta, half-&-half, egg, 1/8 tsp, 1/4 cups of Parmesan salt, & 1/8 tsp pepper.

4. In 2 separate gratin dishes, you have to place a layer of the eggplant slices & then sprinkle with the parmesan, pepper, salt & 1/2 spoon of marinara sauce. After that, add 2nd layer of the eggplant, more pepper & salt, half ricotta mixture, & at last 1 tbsp of the grated parmesan on its top.

5. Place gratins on a baking sheet & bake it for 25-30 mins or till that custard sets & its top is browned.

NUTRITION: Calories: 284 kcal Fat: 5.3 g Protein: 9.7 g Carbs: 24.1 g

12. Zucchini and Eggplant Gratin

Ready in: 20minutes

Servings: 4

Difficulty: Easy

INGREDIENTS

- 1/3 cup cheese

- Olive oil

- 25 oz diced zucchini

- 1 1/3 cup tomato sauce

- 370 crushed eggplant

DIRECTIONS

1. Preheat your non-stick pan on med heat. Then spray both the sides of zucchini & eggplant slices using some oil. Cook it in batches for 2 mins every side / till slightly browned & tender. Shift it to the plate. Then preheat your grill on med-high.

2. Layer 1/3 of zucchini, eggplant, sauce & cheese in the dish. Now repeat with the remaining eggplant, pasta sauce, zucchini & cheese.

3. Grill it for 5 mins / till cheese is melted & lightly browned.

NUTRITION: Calories: 746 kcal Fat: 10.2 g Protein: 10.8 g Carbs: 9.4 g

13. Brown Butter Cauliflower Mash

Ready in: 30 minutes

Servings: 6

Difficulty: Easy

INGREDIENTS

- 2 tbsp butter

- One crushed cauliflower

- Salt to taste

- ½ cup sour cream

- ½ tsp pepper

- 1 tbsp crushed chives

- ¼ cup chopped cheese

DIRECTIONS

1. Fill water in the large oven to depth: 1/4 inch. Now arrange the cauliflower in the oven. Cover it while cooking on med-high heat for 7-10 mins / till tender. Then drain.

2. Process the cauliflower, salt, pepper & sour cream in the food processor for 30 seconds - 1 min / till it's smooth, stop scraping down the sides as needed. Then stir in the Parmesan cheese & chives & place in a bowl.

3. If wanted, put microwave mixture on HIGH for 1-2 mins/ till thoroughly heated, stir at 1-min intervals.

4. Cook the butter in a small but heavy saucepan on med heat, constantly stirring, 4-5 mins / till the butter becomes golden brown. Then remove from the heat & immediately drizzle the butter on cauliflower mix. Garnish, if needed. Serve it immediately.

NUTRITION: Calories: 342 kcal Fat: 10 g Protein: 9 g Carbs: 5 g

14. Homemade Tortillas

Ready in: 30 minutes

Servings: 5

Difficulty: Easy

INGREDIENTS

- 3 tbsp olive oil

- 2 cups flour

- ¾ cups water

- Salt to taste

DIRECTIONS

1. In the large bowl, mix flour & salt. Mix in water & oil. Turn it on the floured surface & knead it 10-12 times. Add some flour/water if desired to make a smooth dough. Then let it rest for 10 mins.

2. Divide the dough into eight pieces. On a lightly floured surface, then roll each piece into a 7-inch circle.

3. Cook the tortillas on med heat till lightly browned, in the cast-iron pan, for 1 min on sides. Serve hot

NUTRITION: Calories: 159 kcal Fat: 5 g Protein: 3 g Carbs: 24 g

15. Red Cabbage Slaw

Ready in: 4 hours 15 minutes

Servings: 6

Difficulty: Difficult

INGREDIENTS

- 1 tbsp sugar

- One crushed Cabbage

- ½ cup mayonnaise

- ½ cup chopped carrot

- ¼ cup chopped cranberries

- 1 tbsp milk

- ¼ cups crushed walnuts

- 1 tbsp vinegar

DIRECTIONS

1. Mix cabbage, mayonnaise, carrot, cranberries, milk, walnuts, sugar, & cider vinegar in the bowl; mix well. Cover it & refrigerate till chilled, almost for 4 hrs.

NUTRITION: Calories: 216 kcal Fat: 18 g Protein: 2.4 g Carbs: 14 g

Chapter 5: Soup Recipes

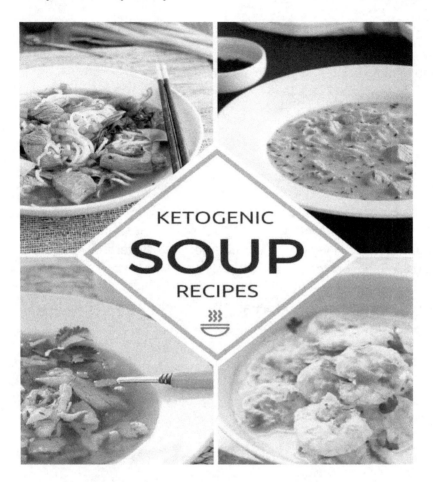

1. Harvest Pumpkin Soup

Ready in: 50 minutes

Servings: 8

Difficulty: Medium

INGREDIENTS

- 2 tbsp chopped pistachios

- 2 tbsp butter

- ½ chopped onion

- One chopped potato

- 4 ½ cups chicken soup

- Salt to taste

- 15 oz pumpkin puree

- ½ cup cream

- Black pepper to taste

- ¼ tsp nutmeg

- ½ cup milk

DIRECTIONS

1. In a cooking pan, mix onions and potatoes with butter for 9 to 11 minutes till the onion become translucent.

2. For fifteen minutes, boil it on low to medium flame.

3. Mix them in pumpkins until it becomes smooth; take salt and paper and the nutmeg to taste.

4. Cook it on high flame until it boils, and boil it for 9 to 11 minutes.

5. Mix it with milk and cream on flame, add salt and paper.

6. Serve it and enjoy it.

NUTRITION: Calories: 185 kcal Fat: 11 g Protein: 6 g Carbs: 17 g

2. Beef Stew

Ready in: 150 minutes

Servings: 4

Difficulty: Difficult

INGREDIENTS

- Two chopped potatoes, baking

- ¼ cup flour

- 1 lb beef

- ¼ tsp pepper

- 5 tsp oil

- 1 cup wine

- 2 tbsp vinegar

- 3 ½ cup beef coup

- One crushed onion

- Two chopped bay leaves

- Salt to taste

- Five chopped carrot

DIRECTIONS

1. Mix flour and pepper the beef and toss.

2. In a pan, heat the oil and put pieces of beef one by 1. Cook it from all sides till brown color.

3. In a pan, mix vinegar and wine and put them into the beef with beef broth and bay leaves. Boiled it until the beef become smooth and soft for about 90 minutes. Put carrots, potatoes, and onion in it and boil it for 25 to 30 minutes.

4. Add water if it dries and flavors it with salt and pepper to taste and enjoy the meal.

NUTRITION: Calories: 494 kcal Fat: 2 g Protein: 35 g Carbs: 54 g

3. Creamy Garlic Bacon Chicken Soup

Ready in: 30 minutes

Servings: 4

Difficulty: Easy

INGREDIENTS

- 2 tbsp crushed parsley

- Four chopped bacon

- Salt to taste

- Six boneless chicken

- Black pepper to taste

- ½ tsp garlic paste

- 8 oz chopped Mushroom

- 1 tsp chopped thyme

- ½ tsp onion powder

- One chopped onion

- ½ tsp sweet paprika

- Three cloves chopped Garlic

- 2/3 cup cream

- ¾ cup chicken soup

DIRECTIONS

1. In a pan, fry diced bacon until it becomes crispy.

2. Bake bacon pieces on the stove and set them on high flame. Flavor chicken thighs with garlic powder, pepper, paprika, salt, thyme, and onion powder.

3. Turn it and bake it from each side for 5 to 7 minutes on each side.

4. Add the onion to a frying pan and fry it for 120 seconds with garlic in it with mushrooms for 20 seconds. Flavor them with salt and pepper to taste and cook it for 6 minutes; mix the chicken broth and mix it with cream and boil for 6 minutes.

5. Add chicken thighs to the front pan and cook it for 6 minutes till the source became thick.

6. Garnish it with bacon and parsley, serve it and enjoy it.

NUTRITION: Calories: 527 kcal Fat: 37 g Protein: 41 g Carbs: 8 g

4. Creamy Chicken Bacon Noodle Soup

Ready in: 45 minutes

Servings: 5

Difficulty: Easy

INGREDIENTS

- 1 oz egg noodles

- Six chopped bacon

- 1 tbsp Butter

- 1 lb chicken breast

- Three chopped ribs Celery

- Black pepper to taste

- One crushed onion

- 6 oz chopped Mushroom

- ½ tsp sliced thyme

- Two cloves chopped garlic

- Salt to taste

- 1 tsp garlic powder

- 4 cups chicken soup

- ½ tsp paprika

101

- 8 oz creamy cheese

- Chopped green onion

- 1 cup cream

- Crushed parsley

DIRECTIONS

1. In a frying pan, cook bacon till it becomes crispy.

2. Spread salt, garlic powdered, and black pepper on chicken breast.

3. Cook bacon and chicken breast for 180 seconds on each side.

4. Add one tablespoon butter to the frying pan; now mix onion, diced shallot, celery, and mushrooms till they become soft. Mix smoked paprika salt dried thyme, black pepper, garlic powder, and garlic, and cook it for 1 minute. Add

5. chicken stock which is 4 cups, and boil them. No mix in it, ramens, and egg noddle.

6. Add chicken and bacon to the pan mix and boiled for 16 minutes; also mix cream 1 cup cheese cubed and heavy cream when everything is fully mixed, then garnishes it with green onion, serve it and enjoy it

NUTRITION: Calories: 399 kcal Fat: 33 g Protein: 51 g Carbs: 47 g

5. Creamy Bacon Mushroom Thyme Chicken

Ready in: 35 minutes

Servings: 4

Difficulty: Medium

INGREDIENTS

- 1 tbsp thyme

- 4 lb boneless chicken

- Six chopped bacon

- 1 tbsp olive oil

- Salt to taste

- 1 tsp garlic powder

- 1 cup cream

- Black pepper to taste

DIRECTIONS

1. In a pan, mix chicken thighs and flavor them with salt and paper.

2. Cook chicken for 60 to 120 seconds till it becomes brown, and bakes them for 21 minutes in the oven until it is cooked.

3. Mix mushrooms with olive oil in a pan; now add thyme, began garlic powder has a cream salt and pepper. Boil it until the sauce becomes thick.

4. Mix chicken with them in the pan and cook it and serve the meal.

NUTRITION: Calories: 741 kcal Fat: 66 g Protein: 31 g Carbs: 6 g

6. Bacon Cheddar Ranch Chicken Noddle Soup

Ready in: 30 minutes

Servings: 5

Difficulty: Easy

INGREDIENTS

- 8 oz chopped cheese

- 1 tbsp olive oil

- 12 oz crushed bacon

- 1 cup crushed onion

- 8 cup chicken soup

- 1 oz Ranch Dressing

- 3 cup noodles

- 4 cups chicken, cooked

- 2 cups heavy cream (half and a half)

- ¼ cup chopped chives

DIRECTIONS

1. In a pan, add bacon pieces and fry until crispy over medium flame with occasional stirring. Drain and set aside.

2. In another pot, heat oil and sauté onions in it for more than five minutes.

3. Pour in chicken stock and let it boil.

4. Add noodles and cook for three minutes.

5. Add ranch dressing and a half and a half and whisk well.

6. Pour the ranch dressing mixture into the pot and mix well.

7. Mix in chicken and cook for few minutes.

8. Use cooked bacon, cheese, and chives for serving.

9. Enjoy it.

NUTRITION: Calories: 439 kcal Fat: 26 g Protein: 33 g Carbs: 19 g

7. Rabbit Stew with Mushrooms

Ready in: 150 minutes

Servings: 4

Difficulty: difficult

INGREDIENTS

- 3 cups chicken soup

- 1 oz porcini Mushroom

- 1 tbsp olive oil

- Three crushed shallots

- Two chopped Garlic

- 1 ½ lb Mushroom

- One rabbit

- 4 tbsp butter

- 2 cups Mushroom water

- 1 tbsp dried thyme

- Salt to taste

- One crushed parsnip

- 2 tbsp crushed parsley

DIRECTIONS

1. Soak the Mushroom in hot water and salt the rabbit pieces. In a hot oven, bake the garlic head drizzled with olive oil for ¾ hour.

2. Cut the rough end of mushrooms and dehydrate the porcini, and save the liquid of the mushrooms.

3. In a pan, release the water in mushrooms by heating them use salt for best results.

4. In a pan, add butter and rabbit pieces and cook it until the pieces became brown.

5. Put the shallots and cook it for 4 minutes, and spread the salt on it also.

6. Now pinch the garlic in the water of Mushroom and mic them.

7. Combine the sherry or wine into the shallots, add mushroom and garlic mixture, and stir them.

8. Finally, add thyme, parsnips, Mushroom, and rabbit pieces, and mix them well. And boil it for 1.5 hours

9. Sever it and enjoy it.

NUTRITION: Calories: 676 kcal Fat: 33.3 g Protein: 79.1 g Carbs: 21.9 g

8. Rabbit Stew

Ready in: 70 minutes

Servings: 5

Difficulty: Medium

INGREDIENTS

- One crushed onion

- 4 Rabbit Legs

- Salt to taste

- 100 g flour

- Black pepper to taste

- 1 tbsp olive oil

- 25 g Butter

- One stick crushed celery

- 11 cup chicken stock

- 200 g mushroom

- One chopped Thyme

DIRECTIONS

1. Mix rabbit legs with a mixture of salt flour.

2. Bake the legs in butter and oil until the brown color is shown.

3. Combine the Mushroom, onion, and celery in a hot pot on medium flame. Combine flour with wine and mix with rabbit legs and also add thyme, chicken stock, and rabbit legs such that legs are merged in it.

4. Boil the mixture for up to 1-hour till tender the legs.

5. Serve It and enjoy the meal.

NUTRITION: Calories: 60 kcal Fat: 21 g Protein: 61 g Carbs: 36 g

9. Lentil and Sausage Soup Spinach Russian salad

Ready in: 3 hours 15 minutes

Servings: 10

Difficulty: Difficult

INGREDIENTS

- ½ lb Italian sausage

- One stalk Celery

- One crushed onion

- 16 oz Dry Lentils

- 1 tbsp garlic paste

- 1 cup chopped carrot

- 15.5 oz chicken soup

- 1 tbsp garlic powder

- 8 cups water

- 28 oz chopped tomatoes

- Two bay leaves

- 1 tbsp Crushed parsley

- ¼ tsp chopped Thyme

- ½ tsp Chopped Oregano

- ¼ tsp Chopped basil

- Salt to taste

- ½ lb pasta

- Black pepper to taste

DIRECTIONS

1. Add sausage to a pan and cook it till brown and mix the onion, celery, sauté, and garlic.

2. Combine carrot, tomatoes, water, chicken broth in lentils.

3. Flavor them with pepper, oregano, thyme, garlic powder, salt, bay leaves, and basil.

4. Boil the mixture for 150 to 180 minutes till lentils become soft. Now add pasta and bake it for 18 to 19 minutes.

NUTRITION: Calories: 353 kcal Fat: 8 g Protein: 18.9 g Carbs: 50.2 g

10. White Chicken Chili

Ready in: 15 minutes

Servings: 6

Difficulty: Easy

INGREDIENTS

- 14.5 oz chicken soup

- One chopped onion

- Two cloves chopped Garlic

- 1 tbsp olive oil

- 1 ½ tsp cumin

- ½ tsp paprika

- ½ tsp chopped coriander

- ¼ tsp Cayenne pepper

- ½ tsp chopped oregano

- Salt to taste

- 7 oz green pepper

- 8 oz cheese

- 15 oz cannellini beans

- One ¼ cup corn

- 2 ½ cup chopped Rotisserie, cooked

- 2 tbsp crushed Cilantro

- 1 tbsp Lemon juice

- Tortilla chips

DIRECTIONS

1. In oil, mix onion and garlic and cook it.

2. Mix cumin, cayenne pepper, green chilies, oregano, chicken broth, and paprika; add the salt and pepper flavor and boil it for 16 minutes.

3. Drain the beans, add them to the blender, process them with broth, and puree until soft and smooth.

4. Mix the cheese and corn with beans and processed beans, mix them, and boil for 9 to 10 minutes. Finally, mix lime juice and cilantro.

5. Serve and enjoy it,

NUTRITION: Calories: 383 kcal Fat: 14 g Protein: 33 g Carbs: 35 g

11. Keto Crab Dip Soup

Ready in: 15 minutes

Servings: 6

Difficulty: Easy

INGREDIENTS

- 1 lb Lump crabmeat

- 1 tbsp ghee

- ¾ cup Chopped Parmesan Cheese

- Tbsp seasoning

- 3 cups milk (Half and Half)

- 8 oz cream cheese

DIRECTIONS

1. in a pan, add butter and cream cheese, whisk, stir and smooth it. Mix parmesan cheese using a blender or mixer until it becomes smooth, softly put crab meat, avoid chunks, and finally, the soup is ready to enjoy.

NUTRITION: Calories: 358 kcal Fat: 27 g Protein: 21 g Carbs: 5 g

12. Tomato Feta soup

Ready in: 30 minutes

Servings: 6

Difficulty: Easy

INGREDIENTS

- 2/3 cup chopped Cheese

- 2 tbsp butter

- 1/3 cup cream

- ¼ cup crushed onion

- 3 cups water

- Two cloves chopped Garlic

- 1 tsp sugar

- Salt to taste

- 1 tsp honey

- Black pepper to taste

- Ten crushed tomatoes

- 1 tsp pesto sauce

- ½ tsp chopped oregano

- 1 tbsp tomato paste

- 1 tsp crushed basil

DIRECTIONS

1. in olive oil, mix onion and cook for 120 seconds, garlic for 1 minute. Now combine tomatoes, water, salt, basil, pepper, oregano, pesto, boil them, and add sweeteners. Bake it for 20 to 25 minutes. Finally, using a blender made it smooth and also mixed cream and cheese in it. Serve and enjoy it.

NUTRITION: Calories: 170 kcal Fat: 13 g Protein: 4 g Carbs: 10 g

13. Creamy Keto Tuscan Soup

Ready in: 17 minutes

Servings: 6

Difficulty: Easy

INGREDIENTS

- 1 cup chopped spinach

- 1 lb sausage

- 1 cup cream

- Two stalks chopped celery

- ¼ cup chopped Garlic

- 3 cup beef soup

- 8 oz cream cheese

- 1 cup red chili

DIRECTIONS

1. In a pan, brown the sausage and break it into pieces. Set sausages aside. In the same pan, add onions and celery and cook until soft add garlic and cook for 3 minutes. Mix sausages back to the pot and add cream cheese and roasted red peppers. Mix until cheeses are melted into meat and vegetables. Stir and add beef stock and bring it to boil. Remove heat and add cream while whisking it. When spinach is soft, and soup is cooked. Remove it from flame and serve

NUTRITION: Calories: 534 kcal Fat: 23 g Protein: 17 g Carbs: 9 g

14. Creamy Tuscan Garlic Tortellini Soup

Ready in: 15 minutes

Servings: 8

Difficulty: Easy

INGREDIENTS

*   2 cups chopped spinach

*   2 tbsp butter

*   9 oz tortellini

*   One chopped onion

*   4 cups chicken soup

*   2 cup chopped chicken, cooked

*   28 oz chopped tomatoes

- Black pepper to taste

- 1 cup cream

- Salt to taste

- 1 tbsp Italian seasoning

- ¼ cup chopped parmesan cheese

DIRECTIONS

1. In a pan, heat the butter and combine onion, and garlic and bake it. Put chicken broth, salt and pepper, diced tomatoes, Italian seasoning, white beans, parmesan cheese, and heavy cream in it and boil it. Combine the chicken, tortellini, and spinach and boil for 12 minutes till it thickens.

NUTRITION: Calories: 397 kcal Fat: 20 g Protein: 21 g Carbs: 34 g

15. Keto Smoked Sausage Cheddar Beer Soup

Ready in: 6 Hours 30 minutes

Servings: 14

Difficulty: Difficult

INGREDIENTS

- 2 cups cheddar Cheese

- 8 oz cheese cream

- 14 oz Beef

- 1 cup cream

- 12 oz beer (extra Beef Soup)

- Black pepper to taste

- 1 cup crushed Carrots

- 1 cup crushed celery

- Salt to taste

- One chopped onion

- 1 tsp Red chili

- Four cloves chopped garlic

DIRECTIONS

1. in cooked, combine celery, salt and pepper, sausage, garlic, beef stock, red pepper flakes, and onion and cook for 3 to 4 hours. Then mix cream, cheddar, and cream cheese. Mix it well using a blender or whisk it well. Add salt and pepper if needed and bake it for more time. Serve and enjoy it.

NUTRITION: Calories: 244 kcal Fat: 17 g Protein: 5 g Carbs: 4 g

Chapter 6: Salad Recipes

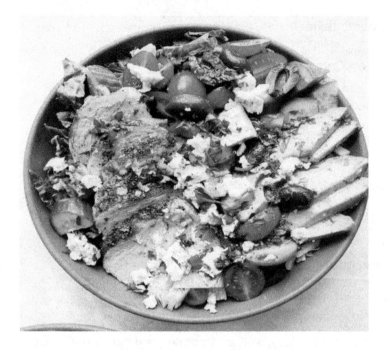

1. Garlic Broccoli

Ready in 5 minutes

Servings: 3

Difficulty: Easy

INGREDIENTS

- 2 tbsp lemon juice

- 1 ½ cup Broccoli florets

- 1 tbsp olive oil

- Black pepper to taste

- 1 tbsp butter

- Three garlic cloves

- salt to taste

DIRECTIONS

1. Boil the broccoli for 1-2 minutes. Drain and keep aside.

2. Take a skillet and heat over medium flame. Put butter and oil in it and fry garlic till it is brown.

3. Now add broccoli.

4. Season with salt and pepper and add lemon juice.

5. Stir well and remove from stove.

6. Serve and enjoy.

NUTRITION: Calories: 111 cal Fat: 8 g Protein: 2 g Carbs: 7 g

2. Creamed Coconut Spinach

Ready in 25 minutes

Servings: 3

Difficulty: Easy

INGREDIENTS

- Black pepper to taste

- 3 tbsp of ghee

- Two shallots

- 20 oz spinach leaves

- 1 tbsp minced ginger

- ½ tsp of cumin

- 2 tbsp of jalapeno chile

- 1 cup of coconut milk

- salt to taste

- 2 tbsp of all-purpose flour

DIRECTIONS

1. Heat ghee in a large Dutch oven and cook spinach for 3-5 minutes. Drain and keep aside to cool. Then chop it.

2. Melt 2 tbsp of ghee in a pan over medium heat. Cook jalapeno, ginger, and shallots for 3-5 minutes. Add cumin, sugar, and flour and cook for 2-3 minutes.

3. Add coconut milk and whisk well.

4. Bring a boil and allow it to simmer for 2-3 minutes.

5. Add chopped spinach.

6. Season with salt and pepper.

7. Serve and enjoy.

NUTRITION: Calories: 139.2 kcal Fat: 9.2 g Protein: 2.6 g Carbs: 12.1 g

3. Creamed Cauliflower

Ready in 10 minutes

Servings: 8

Difficulty: Easy

INGREDIENTS

- Black pepper

- 2 ½ cups Cauliflower

- Three garlic cloves

- 1 tsp of parsley

- One diced onion

- 1/4 cup butter

- ¼ cup all-purpose flour

- 1 cup whole milk

- ½ cup of parmesan cheese

DIRECTIONS

1. Steam, drain and cool the cauliflower.

2. Melt butter in the skillet and add flour. Cook till it forms a paste.

3. Add garlic and onion and cook at high heat.

4. Add milk slowly.

5. Stir continuously till the cream is formed.

6. Season with salt and pepper.

7. Mix the cheese in it and stir till it is melted.

8. Add cauliflower and allow to simmer for 3-5 minutes.

9. If the sauce is too thick, add milk according to the requirement.

10. Garnish with parsley and pepper.

11. Serve and enjoy.

NUTRITION: Calories: 176k cal Fat: 4 g Protein: 4 g Carbs: 7 g

4. Radishes with Herbed Salt and Olive Oil

Ready in: 25 minutes

Servings: 8

Difficulty: Easy

INGREDIENTS

- 1 tsp of salt

- Two garlic clove

- 2tbsp of chopped parsley

- 1 tsp of olive oil

- 2tbsp of chopped chives

- 1tbsp of chopped tarragon leaves

- ½ tsp of peppercorns

- 2tsp of grated lemon zest

- 2 lb of radishes

DIRECTIONS

1. Mix all the ingredients in a large bowl.

2. Season with salt and pepper.

3. Add oil in a separate small bowl.

4. Serve radishes with herbed salt and oil for dipping.

5. Enjoy.

NUTRITION: Calories: 83, Fat: 12 g, Proteins: 1 g, Carbs: 4 g

5. Grilled Asparagus Medley

Ready in: 25 minutes

Servings: 8

Difficulty: Easy

INGREDIENTS

- ¼ tsp of dill weed

- 1 lb asparagus

- 1 cup sliced mushrooms

- 2 cups pepper (Yellow, red, and green)

- ¼ tsp pepper

- One chopped tomato

- 2tbsp of olive oil

- One garlic clove

- 1tsp of parsley

- ½ tsp of salt

- ¼ tsp of lemon pepper

DIRECTIONS

1. Mix vegetables, garlic, and olives in a bowl.

2. Add oil and toss to coat.

3. Sprinkle it with parsley, pepper, salt, and lemon pepper.

4. Toss again well.

5. Grill over medium heat for 20-30 minutes.

6. Stir occasionally.

7. Serve and enjoy.

NUTRITION: Calories: 78 cal Fat: 5 g Protein: 3g Carbs: 8 g

6. Creamy Fennel Sauce

Ready in: 20 minutes

Servings: 6

Difficulty: Easy

INGREDIENTS

- Salt to taste

- 2 cups Cream

- One shallot

- ½ cup White wine

- One garlic clove

- 2 tbsp White flour

- 1 oz cream cheese

- ½ tsp Herbs

- White pepper to taste

- 2 tbsp nutmeg, grated

DIRECTIONS

1. Take a food processor and process chopped shallot and fennel till they are minced completely.

2. Take a pot and melt butter. Add vegetables and cook for 2-5 minutes.

3. Now transfer cooked vegetables to a separate bowl and keep them aside.

4. Melt butter and add flour to it.

125

5. Cook till it becomes golden.

6. Add white wine. Stir continuously.

7. Add cream and cheese and cook till it melts.

8. Return vegetables to pot and mix with sauce, herbs, and nutmeg.

9. Season with salt and pepper. Simmer for 15-20 minutes.

10. Serve and enjoy.

NUTRITION: Calories: 200 cal Fat: 8 g Protein: 10 g Carbs: 20 g

7. Zucchini with Mint

Ready in: 15 minutes

Servings: 4

Difficulty: Easy

INGREDIENTS

- 1 tbsp of mint, chopped

- 12 small zucchini

- 2 Scallions

- 2 tbsp olive oil

- 1 tbsp lemon juice

- Salt to taste

- ½ tbsp of parsley leaf, chopped

DIRECTIONS

1. Cut zucchini lengthwise.

2. Take a skillet and heat olive oil over medium heat.

3. Add scallions and sauté.

4. Add zucchini and salt to taste.

5. When zucchini starts to become golden, then reduce the heat.

6. Add lemon juice and sprinkle mint & parsley.

7. Cook for 1-2 minutes.

8. Serve and enjoy.

NUTRITION: Calories: 125 cal Fat: 8 g Protein: 5 g Carbs: 13 g

8. Warm Crab and Spinach Dip

Ready in: 20 minutes

Servings: 2

Difficulty: Easy

INGREDIENTS

*   2 cups cheddar cheese

*   2tbsp olive oil

*   Two minced garlic cloves

*   1/3 cup chopped onion

- 1 cup cream cheese

- ¼ cup of milk

- 1 cup garlic and herb cheese

- ¼ cup wine

- 2 tsp of Worcestershire sauce

- 1 tbsp of seafood seasoning

- 1/8 tsp of red pepper flakes

- 2 cups chopped spinach

- 2 lb crabmeat

- Tortilla chips

DIRECTIONS

1. Take a skillet and heat over medium flame.

2. Cook onion and garlic for 2-3 minutes.

3. Add cheese and Boursin and stir till melted.

4. Add cream, wine, and milk.

5. Stir continuously.

6. Add seasonings and remaining ingredients.

7. Cook till cheeses are melted.

8. Serve and enjoy.

NUTRITION: Calories: 170 cal Fat: 14g Protein: 9 g Carbs: 2 g

9. Okra Gumbo

Ready in: 15 minutes

Servings: 8

Difficulty: Easy

INGREDIENTS

- 2 Bay leaves

- One chopped onion

- One garlic clove

- One chopped bell pepper

- 8 oz sliced mushrooms

- Two okra

- ½ tsp of file powder

- One diced tomatoes

- 3 tbsp of vegetable oil

- 1 tsp of salt

- 1 tsp of black pepper

- 2 tbsp of all-purpose flour

DIRECTIONS

1. Take pan and heat oil in it over medium heat.

2. Add garlic, bell pepper, and onion.

3. Sauté till tendered.

4. Add mushrooms, tomatoes, tomato paste, file powder, okra, bay leaves, salt & pepper.

5. Stir continuously and cook for 35-40 minutes.

6. Take 2 tbsp of oil in the pan and heat over medium flame. Add flour and cook for 3-5 minutes till it becomes golden.

7. Add roux in okra mixture and cook for 5-10 minutes till it is thickened.

8. Serve and enjoy.

NUTRITION: Calories: 105 cal Fat: 5.5g Protein: 3.2 g Carbs: 12.4 g

10. Stuffed Mushrooms

Ready in: 25 minutes

Servings: 12

Difficulty: Easy

INGREDIENTS

- ¼ tsp of onion powder

- 12 mushrooms

- 1 tbsp minced garlic

- 1 tbsp of vegetable oil

- 1 cup Cream cheese

- ¼ tsp of black pepper

- ¼ cup of parmesan cheese

- ¼ tsp of cayenne pepper

DIRECTIONS

1. Take a large skillet and heat oil.

2. Add garlic and mushrooms' stems.

3. Fry till all the moisture is absorbed. Keep aside and let it cool.

4. Once the mixture is cooled at room temperature, add parmesan and cream cheese, cayenne pepper, onion powder, and black pepper.

5. The mixture should be thick.

6. Fill the mushrooms with the mixture.

7. Arrange the mushrooms in a baking dish.

8. Bake for 15-20 minutes.

9. Serve and enjoy.

NUTRITION: Calories: 88 cal Fat: 8.2 g Protein:2. 7 g Carbs: 1.5 g

11. Seattle Asian Salmon Bowl

Ready in: 10 minutes

Servings: 4

Difficulty: Easy

INGREDIENTS

- One strip Shredded nori

- ½ cup green onions

- 1tbsp sesame seeds (toasted)

- One sliced English cucumber

- 2 cups rice cooked

- 14 oz diced avocado

- ¾ cup Daikon radish

- Salt to taste

- 16 oz salmon

- Black pepper to taste

DIRECTIONS

1. Take a large bowl and mix vinaigrette ingredients.

2. Take a pan and spray with oil.

3. Season the salmon and heat for 4-5 minutes.

4. Divide the hot rice into four bowls.

5. Top with green onions, sesame seeds, cucumbers, sprouts, and avocado.

6. Put salmon in each bowl.

7. Drizzle with vinaigrette.

8. Sprinkle with nori.

9. Serve and enjoy.

NUTRITION: Calories: 395 cal Fat: 5 g Protein:27 g Carbs: 31 g

12. White Bean and Cod Salad

Ready in: 25 minutes

Servings: 3

Difficulty: Easy

INGREDIENTS

- 4 tbsp olive oil

- 300 g white beans

- One diced carrot

- One diced spring onion

- One garlic clove

- Apple cider vinegar as required

- Salt to taste

- Chives as required

DIRECTIONS

1. Take white beans in a pot. Add water till it is covered.

2. Add salt (one pinch) and let it boil for 10-20 minutes.

3. Drain and keep aside.

4. Simmer water in a pot. Put cod in it and cook for 5-10 minutes.

5. Process the garlic in the food processor.

6. Blend oil, vinegar, and garlic. Pour this mixture over cod.

7. Add carrot (shredded) to the beans.

8. Layer the beans on the plate. Divide the cod on top of each plate and sprinkle chives (chopped).

NUTRITION: Calories: 1439 cal Fat: 106.7 g Protein: 68.1 g Carbs: 54.7 g

13. Three Herb Tomato Zucchini Salad

Ready in: 10 minutes

Servings: 4

Difficulty: Easy

INGREDIENTS

- 1 cup Chopped herbs (chive, parsley, basil)

- 2 cups cherry tomatoes

- One sliced shallot

- One zucchini

- 2 tbsp of lemon juice

- 4 tbsp Virgin oil

- 1 tsp Garlic

- 2 tsp Sumac

- Smoked paprika

- 1 tbsp of lemon juice

- salt to taste

- pepper to taste

- 1 Lemon slices round

DIRECTIONS

1. Slice tomatoes and zucchini and put in a large bowl.

2. Slice and soak the shallot in lemon juice. Keep aside.

3. Toss together the chopped herbs in a separate bowl.

4. Mix olive oil, sumac, garlic, salt, lemon juice, pepper, paprika in a large bowl.

5. Add tomatoes and zucchini.

6. Add shallot slices and herbs.

7. Toss well.

8. Garnish with lemon slices.

9. Serve and enjoy.

NUTRITION: Calories: 84 cal Fat: 8.8 g Protein: 0.5 g Carbs: 1.9 g

14. Spinach and Cabbage Slaw

Ready in: 10 minutes

Servings: 6

Difficulty: Easy

INGREDIENTS

- ¼ tsp of dried weed

- 2 cups coleslaw

- ¼ cup red bell pepper

- 2 cups spinach leaves

- ¼ cup ranch salad dressing

DIRECTIONS

1. Mix all the ingredients in a large bowl.

2. Keep in the refrigerator for 10-15 minutes.

3. Serve and enjoy.

NUTRITION: Calories: 35 cal Fat: 20 g Protein: 2 g Carbs: 3 g

15. Avocado Bell Pepper Salad

Ready in: 5 minutes

Servings: 1

Difficulty: Easy

INGREDIENTS

- Two sliced onions

- One diced avocado

- ½ cup cherry tomatoes

- One diced bell pepper

- 2 tbsp of parsley (minced)

- Salt to taste

- 2 tbsp Lemon juice

- Black pepper to taste

DIRECTIONS

1. Mix all the ingredients in a large bowl.

2. Refrigerate for 5-10 minutes.

3. Serve and enjoy.

NUTRITION: Calories: 391 cal Fat: 30 g Protein: 7 g Carbs: 34 g

Chapter 7: Smoothies Recipes

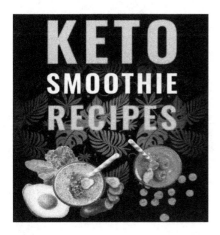

1. Spinach and Avocado Smoothie

Ready in: 3 minutes

Servings: 1

Difficulty: Easy

INGREDIENTS

- 1 cup cold water

- 1 cup chopped mango, frozen

- 2 cups baby spinach

- ½ avocado

- 2 tbsp protein powder

DIRECTIONS

1. Combine mango, spinach, protein powder, avocado, and water in a food processor and blend to get a smooth mixture.

2. Transfer the into the serving glass.

3. Serve and enjoy it.

NUTRITION: Calories: 329 cal Fat: 17 g Protein: 17 g Carbs: 44 g

2. Café Latte

Ready in: 15 minutes

Servings: 4

Difficulty: Easy

INGREDIENTS

- 1 1/3 cup coffee

- 2 cups milk

DIRECTIONS

1. Add milk to the pan and let it boil with constant vigorous stirring to form foam in heating milk.

2. Add coffee to a container and pour in hot water. Stir to dissolve coffee in water.

3. Transfer the coffee into serving cups.

4. Add boiling milk in serving cups and stir

5. Serve and enjoy it.

NUTRITION: Calories: 63 cal Fat: 2.5 g Protein: 4.7 g Carbs: 5.7 g

3. Hot Chocolate

Ready in: 6 minutes

Servings: 4

Difficulty: Easy

INGREDIENTS

- ¼ tsp vanilla extract

- 4 cups milk

- ¼ cup sugar

- ¼ cup cocoa powder

- ½ cup chocolate chips

DIRECTIONS

1. Add sugar with cocoa and milk in a pan and heat on medium flame with constant stirring.

2. Stir in chocolate chips and mix to dissolve them.

3. Mix in vanilla extract and stir well.

4. Serve and enjoy it.

NUTRITION: Calories: 323 cal Fat: 13 g Protein: 9 g Carbs: 42 g

4. Strawberry Protein Smoothie

Ready in: 10 minutes

Servings: 1

Difficulty: Easy

INGREDIENTS

- Five ice cubes

- ½ cup almond milk

- One vanilla protein

- ¾ cup strawberries

- ½ cup greek yogurt

- 1 tsp honey

DIRECTIONS

1. Add all the ingredients into the blender except for ice cubes and blend to get a smooth mixture.

2. In the end, add ice cubes and blend again.

3. Serve and enjoy it.

NUTRITION: Calories: 304 cal Fat: 9.1 g Protein: 31.7 g Carbs: 21.6 g

5. Avocado Raspberry and Chocolate Smoothie

Ready in: 5 minutes

Servings: 1

Difficulty: Easy

INGREDIENTS

- ½ tsp vanilla

- ½ avocado

- 1 tbsp maple syrup

- 1 ½ cups milk

- 1 cup raspberries

- 1 tbsp cocoa powder

DIRECTIONS

1. Add all the ingredients to a food processor and blend to get a smooth, creamy mixture.

2. Serve and enjoy it.

NUTRITION: Calories: 360 cal Fat: 14 g Protein: 10 g Carbs: 55 g

6. Berry Coconut Chia Smoothie

Ready in: 5 minutes

Servings: 2

Difficulty: Easy

INGREDIENTS

- 1 tbsp maple syrup

- 1 cup mixed berries

- One ¼ tbsp coconut milk

- Seven ice cubes

- 1 tbsp chia seeds

- 1 tbsp toasted coconut flakes

DIRECTIONS

1. Soak chia seed in milk and leave it for 20 hours.

2. Add all the ingredients to a food processor and blend to get a smooth, creamy mixture.

3. Serve and enjoy it.

NUTRITION: Calories: 133 kcal Fat: 8 g Protein: 3 g Carbs: 16 g

7. Orange Creamsicle Smoothie

Ready in: 5 minutes

Servings: 2

Difficulty: Easy

INGREDIENTS

- One sliced orange

- One sliced banana

- ½ cup orange juice

- 2 tsp vanilla extract

- ¾ yogurt

DIRECTIONS

1. Add all the ingredients to a food processor and blend to get a smooth, creamy mixture.

2. Serve and enjoy it.

NUTRITION: Calories: 207 kcal Fat: 2 g Protein: 3 g Carbs: 24 g

8. Mint Cocoa Mix

Ready in: 5 minutes

Servings: 53

Difficulty: Easy

INGREDIENTS

- Miniature marshmallows

- 1 cup creamer

- 7 ½ cups chocolate drink

- 2 ½ cups sugar

- 2 oz milk powder

- 25 peppermint candies

DIRECTIONS

1. Add sugar, milk powder, candies, and marshmallows in an airtight bag and shake well.

2. Add cocoa mix and hot milk in a container and stir.

3. Add marshmallows and serve.

NUTRITION: Calories: 259 cal Fat: 9 g Protein: 14 g Carbs: 42 g

9. Chicken Misco Soup

Ready in: 5 minutes

Servings: 2

Difficulty: Easy

INGREDIENTS

- 1 cup spinach

- 2 cups water

- 2 tbsp ginger

- One garlic clove

- 120 sliced chicken

- Two diced mushrooms

- One sliced zucchini

- 2 tbsp miso paste

DIRECTIONS

1. Add water to a pot and let it boil.

2. Stir in garlic and ginger and cook for few minutes.

3. Add chicken pieces and mix. Bring it to simmer for five minutes.

4. Mix in Mushroom and zucchini and cook for five more minutes.

5. Add miso paste and spinach. Cook for one minute.

6. Serve and enjoy it.

NUTRITION: Calories: 134 cal Fat: 3.1 g Protein: 19 g Carbs: 8.5 g

Chapter 8: Breakfast Recipes

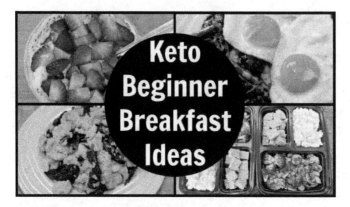

1. Tomato Basil Frittata

Ready in: 35 minutes

Servings: 8

Difficulty: Easy

INGREDIENTS

- ½ cup milk

- 1 cup tomatoes

- ¼ cup chopped onion

- Ten basil leaves

- Ten eggs

- Salt to taste

- Pepper to taste

- 1 cup skimmed mozzarella

DIRECTIONS

1. Add milk, pepper, salt, and eggs to a bowl and beat it.

2. Mix half of the cheese into the above mixture and place it aside.

3. Take a non-stick skillet, spray it with cooking oil and preheat it.

4. Add chopped onion, and cook them for 3 minutes.

5. Cut tomatoes into slices and add them to the pan.

6. Pour the mixture of egg into a pan and cook it for about 4 mins.

7. By using a spatula, pull the edges inward so that it is thoroughly cooked.

8. Repeat this 4 to 5 times.

9. Stop heating the pan.

10. On the top, place basil leaves and add the remaining cheese.

11. Place skillet into a preheated oven at 375°C for 15 minutes.

12. Then cool it for 5 mins.

13. Serve and enjoy it.

NUTRITION: Calories: 129 cal Fat: 8 g Protein: 11 g Carbs: 35 g

2. Coconut Pudding

Ready in: 25 mins

Servings: 4

Difficulty: Easy

INGREDIENTS

- ¼ cup sugar

- Two egg yolks

- 1 tsp coconut extract

- 2 cups coconut milk

- 2tpsp butter

- 2tpsp corn starch

DIRECTIONS

1. Combine all the ingredients in a pan and cook over medium flame.

2. Cook the mixture for 5 to 8 minutes, till it is thickened.

3. Pour the pudding into a bowl and refrigerate it.

NUTRITION: Calories: 382 cal Fat: 32.1 g Protein: 3.7 g Carbs: 23.8 g

3. Coconut Omelet

Ready in: 15 minutes

Servings: 2

Difficulty: Easy

INGREDIENTS

- 1/3 cup grated coconut

- Four eggs

- One chopped green chili

- One chopped onion

- Salt as required

- Few coriander leaves

DIRECTIONS

1. Combine all the ingredients in a mixing bowl.

2. Pour this mixture into a wok.

3. Cook both sides properly.

4. Serve and enjoy Coconut Omelet.

NUTRITION: Calories: 117 cal Fat: 9 g Protein: 7 g Carbs: 4 g

4. Garlic Butter Keto Spinach

Ready in: 10 mins

Servings: 2

Difficulty: Easy

INGREDIENTS

- ¼ tsp black pepper

- 1tbsp butter

- ¼ tsp salt

- 1tbsp chopped garlic

- 10-12 oz. leaves of spinach

DIRECTIONS

1. Melt the butter in a pan over medium heat.

2. Sauté garlic in it for 2 mins and then add diced spinach.

3. Add salt as required and sauté for 3-4 mins over medium heat.

4. Cover the pan with a lid for few minutes.

5. Sauté it, till the water released by spinach evaporates.

6. Turn off the flame and serve it.

NUTRITION: Calories: 70 kcal Fat: 7 g Protein: 1.5 g Carbs: 3 g

5. Cranberry Apple Oatmeal

Ready in: 20 minutes

Servings: 2

Difficulty: Easy

INGREDIENTS

- ½ cup walnuts, chopped

- 2 cups water

- Salt to taste

- One diced apple

- ¼ tsp nutmeg, ground

- ½ cup cranberries, fresh

- ¼ cup sugar

- 1 cup oats (quick-cooking)

- ½ tsp cinnamon, ground

DIRECTIONS

1. Take a bowl and mix cranberries, apple, and water in it, and boil the mixture.

2. Cook it for 6 mins, till the apple becomes tender and the cranberries burst.

3. Add sugar, nutmeg, oats, salt, and cinnamon into the above mixture.

4. Cook the mixture for 3 to 4 mins with continuous stirring.

5. Turn off the flame when oatmeal thickens.

6. Garnish with walnuts and enjoy it.

NUTRITION: Calories: 500 cal Fat: 22 g Protein: 10 g Carbs: 71 g

6. Turkey Omelet

Ready in: 10 minutes

Servings: 1

Difficulty: Easy

INGREDIENTS

- One slice of shredded cheese

- Two eggs

- 3 tsp chopped green peppers

- ¼ cup evaporated milk

- 4 tsp tomato sauce

- 1/3 cup chopped turkey, cooked

- Salt as required

- Pepper as required

- 3 tsp chopped onions

- 2 tsp butter

DIRECTIONS

1. Take a bowl, add evaporated milk, pepper, salt, egg, and beat it.

2. Mix tomato sauce, green onion, green pepper, and turkey in a separate bowl.

3. Take a pan, melt butter over medium flame and add egg mixture to it.

4. Cook it without stirring.

5. Now turn it with the spatula and cook without breaking it.

6. Spread turkey mixture and cheese over it.

7. Fold the Omelet and serve it.

NUTRITION: Calories: 452.6 cal Fat: 29.4 g Protein: 4 g Carbs: 11.4 g

7. Vanilla Pumpkin Bread

Ready in: 60 minutes

Servings: 2

Difficulty: MEDIUM

INGREDIENTS

- 1 tsp cinnamon, ground

- Five eggs

- 2 tsp salt

- One ¼ cup canola oil

- 1 tsp baking soda

- 15 oz. pumpkin

- 2 cups flour(all-purpose)

- 3 oz. vanilla pudding

- 2 cups sugar

DIRECTIONS

1. In a bowl, add pumpkin, oil, egg, and beat till the mixture becomes smooth.

2. Add remaining ingredients and again beat it.

3. Pour the batter into the pan and bake it for 45 mins at 325°.

4. Cool it, and then enjoy.

NUTRITION: Calories: 150 cal Fat: 8 g Protein: 2 g Carbs: 20 g

8. Zucchini Omelet

Ready in: 15 minutes

Servings: 2

Difficulty: Easy

INGREDIENTS

- 3tpsp cheese, shredded

- ½ cup zucchini, sliced

- Pepper as required

- 1/8 tsp salt

- Two onions, sliced

- 1/8 tsp thyme, dried

- 2tbsp butter

- 3tbsp water

- Three eggs

- ¼ cup tomato, chopped

DIRECTIONS

1. Sauté onion and zucchini in butter.

2. Mix all ingredients in a bowl and pour it.

3. Cook it over medium flame.

4. Top egg mixture with cheese and tomatoes.

5. Broil it for 3 mins and serve it.

NUTRITION: Calories: 258 cal Fat: 21 g Protein: 13 g Carbs: 4 g

9. Leek Frittata

Ready in: 30 minutes

Servings: 4

Difficulty: Easy

INGREDIENTS

- 1 oz. shredded cheese

- ¼ cup milk

- Eight beaten eggs

- One minced garlic clove

- 1tbsp flour, all-purpose

- One sliced leek

- ¼ tsp salt

- 1tbsp oil

- ¼ tsp pepper

DIRECTIONS

1. Whisk salt, eggs, flour, pepper, cheese, and milk in a bowl.

2. Take a pan, add oil, and cook leek in it for 2-3 mins.

3. Then add garlic and cook it for 20 sec.

4. Now add the egg mixture in it, with stirring.

5. Cook it over low flame for 6-7 mins.

6. Bake it at 350°F for 12-13 mins.

7. Cut it into wedges and serve it.

NUTRITION: Calories: 230 cal Fat: 15.1 g Protein: 16 g Carbs: 7 g

10. Simple Breakfast Casserole

Ready in: 1 hour 10 minutes

Servings: 12

Difficulty: Difficult

INGREDIENTS

- ½ tsp black pepper, ground

- 8 cups hash browns, frozen

- Cooking spray

- 1 cup milk

- 16 oz. ham, cubed

- 1 tsp salt

- 12 eggs

- 8 oz. shredded cheese

DIRECTIONS

1. Take a bowl and mix ham, cheese, and potatoes in it.

2. Whisk milk, salt, pepper, and eggs in a separate bowl.

3. Spray the baking dish with oil and pour both mixtures in it.

4. Bake it in a preheated oven at 350 F for 60 minutes.

5. Serve and enjoy it.

NUTRITION: Calories: 208 kcal Fat: 9.8 g Protein: 17.3 g Carbs: 13.2 g

Chapter 9: Lunch Recipes

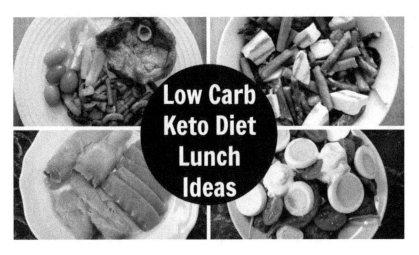

1. Coriander Duck with Sweet Potato Sauce

Ready in: 180 minutes

Servings: 4

Difficulty: Difficult

INGREDIENTS

- Black pepper to taste

- 2 lb. potatoes

- 6 lb. duck

- Salt to taste

- Two chopped onion

- 5 tsp seed oil

- One chopped carrot

- One chopped celery

- Two parsnips

- 8 cups duck stock

- Two lemon

- 1 tbsp coriander seeds

- 1 tbsp lemon juice

- One chili

- 1 tbsp crushed parsley

- 1/8 oz ginger

DIRECTIONS

1. Add water and potatoes to the blender.

2. Transfer the puree to the bowl.

3. Rub meat with seasoning.

4. Heat oil in the skillet and cook meat.

5. Mix in celery, onions, and carrot and let them cook for few minutes.

6. Pour in broth and let it simmer for one hour.

7.   Stir in parsnips and cook for another half an hour.

8.   Strain away the solid part and cook to thicken the solution.

9.   Roast the coriander for half a minute and add to the solution.

10.   Bake the parsnips in the oven for 15 minutes.

11.   Now prepare the potato sauce. Boil the potato juice and mix in lemon zest.

12.   Add lemon juice, ginger, and chili, and cook for a minute.

13.   Serve and enjoy it.

NUTRITION: Calories: 248 kcal Fat: 7.2 g Protein: 41.9 g Carbs: 1.5 g

2. Skillet Chicken with Mushrooms and Pepper

Ready in: 30 minutes

Servings: 4

Difficulty: Easy

INGREDIENTS

- 4 tbsp Avocado oil

- ½ tsp chopped thyme

- 1 lb. boneless chicken

- ½ tsp chopped rosemary

- ½ tsp salt

- ½ tsp chopped oregano

- One chopped red chili

- ¼ tsp pepper

- 8 oz chopped white Mushroom

- One chopped yellow pepper

- ½ cup white wine

- 1 tsp garlic

DIRECTIONS

1. Drizzle oil over chicken.

2. Add salt, rosemary, thyme, pepper, and oregano, and coat chicken in it.

3. Heat oil in pan and cook meat from both sides for five minutes.

4. Sauté mushrooms with pepper and garlic in heated oil for five minutes.

5. Add chicken and cook for ten more minutes.

6. Serve and enjoy it.

NUTRITION: Calories: 297 kcal Fat: 17.4 g Protein: 27.9 g Carbs: 5.8 g

3. Chili Pork chops

Ready in 30 minutes

Servings: 4

Difficulty: Easy

INGREDIENTS

- 2 tbsp honey

- Four pork chops

- 6 tbsp chili sauce

- Salt to taste

- 2 tbsp soy sauce

- 1 tbsp olive oil

- Black pepper to taste.

- 200g carrots

- 200g zucchini

- One minced bulb of garlic

- One diced onion

DIRECTIONS

1. Combine all the ingredients of marination and add chops. Set them aside for half an hour.

2. Cook the chops from both sides in the skillet.

3. Heat oil in another skillet and cook courgette, garlic, onion, and carrot for few minutes.

4. Serve and enjoy it.

NUTRITION: Calories: 605 kcal Fat: 12 g Protein: 40 g Carbs: 69 g

4. Stuffed Tomatoes with Lamb, dill, and Rice

Ready in: 65 minutes

Servings: 4

Difficulty: Medium

INGREDIENTS

- Two bulbs garlic

- Four beefsteak Tomatoes

- ½ tsp sugar

- 4 tbsp olive oil

- 1 tsp cinnamon

- 200 g chopped lamb

- 50g rice

- 2 tbsp tomato sauce

- 4 tbsp diced dill

- 1 cup chicken soup

- 1 tbsp diced mint

- 2 tbsp diced parsley

DIRECTIONS

1. He toils in the skillet and sautés onion, garlic for ten minutes.

2. Add lamb with tomato and cinnamon.

3. Add stock, tomato juice, and rice, and let it boil.

4. Add herbs and mix.

5. Fill tomatoes with the mixture and bake in the preheated oven at 350 Fahrenheit for 30 minutes.

6. Serve and enjoy it.

NUTRITION: Calories: 300 kcal Fat: 19 g Protein: 14 g Carbs: 21 g

5. Turkish lamb and dill – Infused bulgur

Ready in: 20 minutes

Servings: 2

Difficulty: Easy

INGREDIENTS

- 1 tsp sumac

- 1 1/3 cherry Tomatoes

- 130 g wheat

- 80 g yogurt

- 10 g dill

- 250g lamb Mince

- 3 tbsp harissa paste

- One bulb garlic

- Salt to taste

- 2 tbsp oil

DIRECTIONS

1. Heat oil and add lamb and salt.

2. Cook for five minutes.

3. Stir in bulgur and pour in water. Cook for ten minutes.

4. Stir in tomatoes. Let it cook.

5. In a bowl, add yogurt and garlic along with pepper, salt, and oil. Whisk well.

6. Add pasta in boiling water with salt and sugar.

7. The harissa paste is ready.

8. Cook the pasta in the skillet for three minutes.

9. Fry dill and onions and blend them with bulgur.

10. Serve and enjoy it.

NUTRITION: Calories: 2490 kcal Fat: 24.9 g Protein: 36.5 g Carbs: 60 g

6. Lamb Cauliflower and Coconut Curry

Ready in: 45 minutes

Servings: 4

Difficulty: Medium

INGREDIENTS

- One sliced carrot

- 1 ½ tbsp olive oil

- 500g lamb Mince

- ½ slice onion

- 1 ½ cups cauliflower

- 2 tsp sliced ginger

- Two slice bulb garlic

- 3 tsp coriander

- 3 tsp cumin

- One bay leaf

- 2 tsp gram masala

- ½ cup water

- ½ cup coconut milk

- 2 tbsp coriander

- 1 ½ cups white Rice

DIRECTIONS

1. Heat one tbsp oil in a huge pot over high warmth. Add the sheep and earthy colored well, separating pieces with a wooden spoon.

2. Return container to high warmth and add remaining oil and carrot. Cook for 3 mins or until the carrot starts to brown. Add cauliflower and cook for a further 3-5 mins until cauliflower starts to the brown season with salt and pepper.

3. Add onion, garlic, and ginger, cook for around 2 mins. Decrease warmth to med at that point, add cumin, coriander, garam masala, and cove leaf and cook for a further 2 mins, mixing continually.

4. Return sheep to the dish and add coconut milk and water, and stew for around 10 mins, scratching the lower part of the container until the fluid has decreased—season to taste.

5. Then, cook rice as directed

6. To serve, split rice between 4 serving bowls, spoon over the lamb curry, and with coriander, garnish it.

NUTRITION: Calories: 64.9 kcal Fat: 30.7 g Protein: 33.5 g Carbs: 3.3 g

7. Glazed Pork Ribs with Green Beans

Ready in: 90 minutes

Servings: 5

Difficulty: difficult

INGREDIENTS

- 4 tbsp syrup

- 2 kg pork ribs

- 2 tbsp soy sauce

- 2 tbsp vinegar

- 400 g beans

- 1 tbsp chopped chili

- Salt to taste

- 2 tbsp butter

DIRECTIONS

1. Heat the oven to 400 Fahrenheit on both the upper and lower shelves.

2. Rinse the ribs, pat them dry, and break them into 2-rib portions. Combine the maple syrup, mustard, soy sauce, and chili powder in a mixing cup. Coat the ribs in the marinade and roast for about 1 hour in a preheated oven. Cover the ribs with aluminum foil if they tend to brown too easily.

3. Rinse the beans and rinse them—Blanch for 8 mins or until al dente in hot, salted water. Drain thoroughly. Separate the ingredients into tiny packets and bind them together with chives. Toss in melted butter.

4. Serve the ribs with the beans.

NUTRITION: Calories: 451 kcal Fat: 21.1 g Protein: 27.8 g Carbs: 39.9 g

8. Philly Cheesesteak

Ready in: 28 minutes

Servings: 4

Difficulty: Easy

INGREDIENTS

- 1 lb steak

- 1/2 tsp salt

- 1/2 tsp Black pepper

- One chopped onion

- Eight slices of provolone cheese

- Four diced Hoagie Rolls

- 2 Tbsp butter

- 2 tbsp garlic

- 3 Tbsp mayonnaise

DIRECTIONS

1. Slice the rolls and cut the onions into small dices.

2. Mix 2-3 tbsp of butter and garlic in a small bowl. Spread this over sliced rolls.

3. Take a skillet and toast the buns till brown.

4. Heat a small amount of oil in the pan and sauté oil onions (diced). Once caramelized, transfer them to a bowl.

5. Put the sliced steak in la, cool for some minutes, and then season with salt and pepper. Stir till the steaks are fully cooked with onions.

6. Top the steaks with cheese.

7. Turn off the stove. The cheese will melt with heat.

8. Spread a layer of mayo and place the bun on each portion.

9. Scrape the beef using a spatula in the bun.

10. Serve and enjoy.

NUTRITION: Calories: 732 Cal Fat: 44 g Protein: 43 g Carbs: 40 g

9. Steak Fajitas Recipe

Ready in: 25 minutes

Servings: 3-4

Difficulty: Easy

INGREDIENTS

- 2 lb sliced sirloin

- One red pepper

- One yellow pepper

- One med onion

- 3 tbsps olive oil

- 1 tbsp lime juice

- 1/2 tsp black pepper

- 1/2 tsp chili powder

- 1 tsp cumin

- pinch cayenne pepper

- 1/2 tsp Kosher salt

- 2 tbsp garlic

- Seven tortillas

DIRECTIONS

1. Put the steak in a plastic bag.

2. Put onions and peppers in a separate bag and add some lime juice, olive oil, cumin, chili powder, salt, and pepper.

3. Shake well.

4. Put some of the marinades over steaks, some over vegetables, and reserve the remaining for use while cooking.

5. Take a large skillet and heat it over medium flame.

6. Put vegetables in the skillet and cook till they are tendered and becomes crispy.

7. Pour the vegetables on a plate.

8. Put steaks in the skillet and cook for 5-10 minutes.

10. Now add vegetables along with the remaining reserved marinade into the skillet.

11. Serve and enjoy.

NUTRITION: Calories: 380 Cal Fat: 16 g Protein: 35 g Carbs: 19 g

10. Pepper Steak Stir Fry

Ready in: 30 minutes

Servings: 5

Difficulty: Easy

INGREDIENTS

- 1 tbsp oil

- One bell pepper (green and red)

- 1 1/4 lb sliced steak

- 2 tsp garlic

- 1 tsp ginger

- Salt & pepper

- 1/4 cup of soy sauce

- 1 1/2 tbsp sugar

- 1 1/2 tbsp cornstarch

DIRECTIONS

1. Take a large pan and heat some olive oil over medium heat.

2. Put peppers and cook for 5 minutes or till tender. After it, put the peppers on the plate.

3. Season the steak with salt and pepper.

4. Increase the heat and cook the steaks in the pan for 5-10 minutes or be browned.

5. Add some garlic and ginger and cook for a further 1 minute.

6. Place the steaks in the pan with pepper.

7. Take a small bowl and mix the sauce, water, sugar, and cornstarch.

8. Pour the sauce on the steaks' mixture. Bring it to simmer and cook for 3-4 minutes.

9. Serve and enjoy.

NUTRITION: Calories: 277 Cal Fat: 10 g Protein: 32 g Carbs: 11 g

11. Easy Balsamic Chicken

Ready in: 20 minutes

Servings: 4

Difficulty: Easy

INGREDIENTS

- One sliced onion

- 2 tsp olive oil

- 1 1/2 lb chicken boneless

- 3/4 tsp kosher salt

- 1/2 tsp black pepper

- 1/3 cup of balsamic vinegar

- 1/3 cup chicken broth

DIRECTIONS

1. Take a pan and heat oil over medium heat.

2. Add onion and cook till they give a brownish look and become soft.

3. Use salt and pepper to season the chicken strips.

4. Add the chicken to the same pan.

5. Cook till the chicken becomes brown for 5-10 minutes.

6. Add some vinegar & chicken broth.

7. Cook till the chicken is reduced by 1/2.

8. Serve and enjoy.

NUTRITION: Calories: 349 Cal Fat: 9 g Protein: 54 g Carbs: 10 g

12. Balsamic Pork with Olives

Ready in: 20 minutes

Servings: 1

Difficulty: Easy

INGREDIENTS

- 1 tsp mustard

- 3 tbsp olive oil

- 3 tbsp vinegar

- Four boneless crushed pork loin

- Two chopped bulbs of garlic

- ½ cup crush basil

- ½ cup sliced olives

DIRECTIONS

1. Combine vinegar, garlic, oil, and mustard.

2. Rub meat with pepper and salt.

3. Drizzle vinegar and set aside.

4. Heat oil in pan and cook meat for five minutes from each side.

NUTRITION: Calories: 487 kcal Fat: 41 g Protein: 27 g Carbs: 2 g

13. Mushroom and Beef Rice

Ready in: 35 minutes

Servings: 5

Difficulty: Medium

INGREDIENTS

- 2 tbsp oil

- 1 lb. Beef

- 8 oz chopped Mushrooms

- One onion

- Three bulbs chopped garlic

- ½ cup cream

- ¼ cup beef soup

- 1 tsp salt

- 2 tbsp soy sauce

- 1 tsp chopped herbs

- 3 cups cooked rice

- Black pepper to taste

DIRECTIONS

1. Heat a skillet to med-high warmth. Add oil, garlic, and onions. Cook. Add meat and mushrooms. Cook until meat and mushrooms are seared, around 10 mins.

2. Add hamburger stock, hefty cream, Worcestershire, dried spices, ocean salt, and dark pepper. Stew for around 5 mins or until everything is consolidated.

NUTRITION: Calories: 318 kcal Fat: 20 g Protein: 12 g Carbs: 20 g

14. Easy Mushroom Rice

Ready in: 65 minutes

Servings: 4

Difficulty: Medium

INGREDIENTS

- oz beep soup

- 1 cup rice

- 10.5 oz onion soup

- ¼ cup butter

- 4 oz chopped mushrooms

DIRECTIONS

1. Preheat the oven to 350 Fahrenheit.

2. In an 8x8 inch casserole dish, combine the rice, onion soup, beef broth, mushrooms, and butter.

3. Cover and roast for 60 mins in a preheated oven.

NUTRITION: Calories: 336 kcal Fat: 13 g Protein: 9.1 g Carbs: 45.4 g

Chapter 10: Dinner Recipes

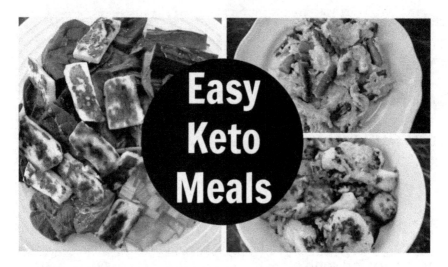

1. Fish Foil Packets with Pesto and Tomatoes

Ready in: 30 minutes

Servings: 2

Difficulty: Easy

INGREDIENTS

- 2 tbsp chopped onion

- Two pieces of white Fish

- 2 tsp fish masala

- 1 tbsp olive oil

- ¼ cup basil pesto pasta

- ¼ cup chopped grape tomatoes

- Lemon juice

DIRECTIONS

1. Take out fish from the store refrigerator, dry it, and rinse both sides with olive oil.

2. Heat grill.

3. Do not wait for grill heating; do other chores like make small pieces of tomatoes and slices of onion.

4. Make sure the aluminum foil is ready and rinse it with olive oil.

5. The major work is to place fish pieces on squared aluminum foil; keep the rule in mind one piece over one square foil, then put the mixture of onion and tomatoes on each piece.

6. By folding foil around fish Cook it on the grill, and do not turn fish while cooking.

7. Cook it for 12-15 minutes; however, time can vary depending upon the thickness of fish or how crusty you want to make it.

8. In the oven, it can be cooked within 15 minutes at 450F

NUTRITION: Calories: 599 kcal Fat: 33 g Protein: 69 g Carbs: 8 g

2. Spicy Red Snapper

Ready in: 45 minutes

Servings: 4

Difficulty: Medium

INGREDIENTS

- 6 oz red Snapper

- 2 tbsp olive oil

- Two cloves chopped garlic

- One sliced of onion

- ½ tbsp chopped red chili

- 14.5 oz stewed tomatoes

- 1 tbsp chopped capers

- Salt to taste

- ½ cup wine

- Black pepper to taste

DIRECTIONS

1. Preferably use the skillet to prepare this recipe. Add some olive oil to it & heat it. Other ingredients like garlic, onion, red pepper and capers also add and heat until onions are soft.

2. Add tomatoes with juice and wine. Now keep the pressure of heat low and stir continuously while cooking.

3. Add snapper fillets in the sauce while it becomes thick. Now cook it for 15-20 minutes at low heat.

NUTRITION: Calories: 297 kcal Fat: 9.4 g Protein: 36 g Carbs: 10.6 g

3. Maryland Crab Cake

Ready in: 55 minutes

Servings: 4

Difficulty: Medium

INGREDIENTS

- 2 tbsp butter

- One egg

- 1 tbsp Dried Parsley

- ¼ cup Mayonnaise

- 2 tsp Mustard

- 1 tsp bay seasoning

- 2 tsp sauce

- 1 tsp Lemon juice

- 1 lb lump crab meat

- Salt to taste

- 2/3 cups cracker Crumbs

DIRECTIONS

1. Combine all the ingredients in a bowl except for crab meat and mix well.

2. Add crab meat and toss to coat it.

3. Place it in the fridge to marinate for more than two hours.

4. Bake in a preheated oven at 450 Fahrenheit for 30 20 minutes.

5. Serve and enjoy it.

NUTRITION: Calories: 299 kcal Fat: 14 g Protein: 32 g Carbs: 9 g

4. Buttered Cod

Ready in: 15 minutes

Servings: 5

Difficulty: Easy

INGREDIENTS

- 1 tbsp parsley

- 1 ½ lb Cod

- ¼ tsp garlic powder

- 6 tbsp butter

- Salt to taste

- ¾ tsp paprika

- Black pepper to taste

- Six slices of lemon

DIRECTIONS

1. To make buttered cod, first mix garlic powder, salt, black pepper, and paprika in a small bowl.

2. Make small pieces of cod. Rinse and pat dry. Then using a seasoning mixture, rinse all sides of codpieces.

3. Take a large skillet, add 2tbsp of butter and melt it at low or medium heat. Now add codpieces and cook for about 2-4 minutes.

4. Now turn over the cod, add four tablespoons of butter on the top of the cod, and heat it for 3 to 4 minutes until butter is completely melted. Make sure it is not overcooked.

5. Now rinse these codpieces with lemon juice and serve it.

NUTRITION: Calories: 1031 kcal Fat: 41 g Protein: 156 g Carbs: 3 g

5. Spinach Octopus

Ready in: 72 minutes

Servings: 2

Difficulty: Difficult

INGREDIENTS

- ½ cup wine

- One crushed onion

- One bay leaf

- Three cloves chopped Garlic

- 1 ½ tsp Spanish paprika

- 1 tbsp olive oil

- Salt to taste

Octopus

- 2 tbsp olive oil

- 1 lb Spanish octopus

Sauce

- 1 tbsp lemon juice

- 1/3 cups braising liquid

- Salt to taste

- 1 tbsp olive oil

- Black pepper to taste

DIRECTIONS

1. Different ingredients used for this recipe are sliced onion, garlic pieces, bay leaf, paprika, and salt. Add all these elements along with 1 tbsp of olive oil in a saucepan and cook them at moderate heat. Stir continuously until the onion becomes soft. White wine will be added to make the braising liquid.

2. Now is time for transferring octopus in braising fluid, cover it, and cook for at least 20 minutes. Then turn over octopus and reduce heat and cook for another 40-45 minutes at low heat.

3. Now remove it from the heat and put it in a large bowl. Soak it in braising liquid. And cool it by placing it on an icy bowl.

4. When it becomes cool, cover it and place it in the refrigerator to freeze it for 2 hours.

5. Now take a paper towel and remove purple skin from it. Make its 3-4 pieces and rinse it with olive oil.

6. Now let's make the sauce. For this, add braising liquid to a saucepan and boil it. Then remove solid material from it, pour it in a mixing bowl, and cool it for 10 minutes. Add fresh lemon juice, olive oil, parsley, table salt, and pepper in it and stir. The serving sauce is ready.

7. Now transfer octopus on a grill that is preheated. Cook it for 3-4 minutes and then turn it and cook the other side. Now transfer it in a platter.

8. Make diagonal slices of octopus pour braising liquid on the top. Now it is ready to serve.

NUTRITION: Calories: 513 kcal Fat: 29.7 g Protein: 35.1 g Carbs: 15 g

6. Keto Zucchini Slice

Ready in: 70 minutes

Servings: 8

Difficulty: Difficult

INGREDIENTS

- 2 1/2 cheese, ricotta

- ½ cup butter

- 2 ½ cup diced bacon

- 1 tbsp olive oil

- Two chopped onions

- 1 cup cream

- 12 eggs

- 1 cup almond meal

- ½ basil, diced

- 5 cup shredded zucchini

- 1 cup shredded cheese, cheddar

DIRECTIONS

1. In the pan, heat oil on a high flame.

2. Heat the bacon & onion for about 5 minutes, stirring frequently, or until crispy.

3. In a separate dish, stir together the milk and eggs.

4. Combine the grated cheese, basil, pork, zucchini, almond meal, and the leftover butter in a mixing bowl.

5. Pour this mixture into the pan that has been packed.

6. Dollop any ricotta on top.

7. Bake in a preheated oven at 400 Fahrenheit 45 minutes, or until golden and solid to the touch.

8. Serve warm or cool, cut into rectangles.

NUTRITION: Calories: 76 kcal Fat: 6 g Protein: 8 g Carbs: 2 g

7. Keto Taco Shells

Ready in: 35 minutes

Servings: 4

Difficulty: Easy

INGREDIENTS

- ½ tsp salt

- ½ cup spinach leaves

- 1/3 cup almond meal

- Two eggs

- 2 tsp psyllium husk

DIRECTIONS

1. In the heatproof dish, position the spinach. To shield, pour hot water over the top. To blanch, set aside about 5 minutes.

2. Place the spinach in the food processor's tank.

3. Combine the psyllium husk, almond meal, eggs, and salt in a mixing bowl.

4. Blend until fully smooth. ¼ of this mixture should be placed on one of these ready baking trays. To create a 15cm shell, spread with a cranked spatula.

5. To make four rings, repeat with the remaining mixture.

6. Bake in the preheated oven at 350 Fahrenheit for 10 minutes or until the center is firm.

7. To make a taco, use a spatula to move circles between spaces of an upraised non-stick muffin tray.

8. Allow cooling slowly before serving.

9. Top with your preferred taco filling.

NUTRITION: Calories: 171 kcal Fat: 13.6 g Protein: 10.6 g Carbs: 1 g

8. Keto Fish and Chips

Ready in: 45 minutes

Servings: 5

Difficulty: Medium

INGREDIENTS

Tartar sauce

- 4 tbsp dill pickle

- ¾ cup mayonnaise

- ½ tbsp curry powder

Chips

- Salt to taste

- 1 ½ lb rutabaga

- Pepper to taste

Fish

- 1 tsp salt

- 1 ½ lb white fish

- 1 cup almond flour

- Two eggs

- 1 cup grated cheese, parmesan

- 1 tsp onion powder

- 1 tsp paprika powder

- 2 cups oil for frying

- ¼ tsp pepper

- One lemon for serving

DIRECTIONS

1. To make the tartar sauce, whisk together all of the ingredients. Refrigerate as you finish the remainder of the bowl.

2. Preheat oven around 400 Fahrenheit.

3. Slice the rutabaga into tiny chips after peeling it.

4. Brush your chips with the oil and sprinkle pepper and salt, and put them on a parchment-lined baking sheet.

5. Considering the thickness of chips, bake for almost 30 minutes or till golden brown.

6. Prepare your fish as rutabaga is frying. In a mixing cup, crack all eggs and whisk them with the fork until the yolks are separated, and the eggs are mixed and frothy.

7. Combine parmesan cheese, almond flour, and seasonings on a pan.

8. Cut your fish in bite-sized portions and coat only with an almond flour mixture. Dip in beaten shells, then powder in almond coating again.

9. In the large saucepan, heat the oil.

10. Remove the pan from the fire and cover it with the lid.

11. Fry your fish for about 3 minutes on either side or until golden brown on both sides and cooked through.

12. Serve with tartar sauce and fried rutabaga fries.

NUTRITION: Calories: 1012 kcal Fat: 74 g Protein: 10.6 g Carbs: 6 g

9. Instant Pot Eggs En Cocotte

Ready in: 5 minutes

Servings: 6

Difficulty: Easy

INGREDIENTS

- 6 tbsp shredded cheese, parmesan

- 1 tbsp butter

- Six eggs

- 6 tsp heavy cream

- Black pepper to taste

DIRECTIONS

1. One teaspoon of heavy cream swirled around in each ramekin to cover the rim.

2. In each ramekin, crack one shell.

3. Then sprinkle cheese on top of each egg.

4. Finally, season the cheese with black pepper. You can do as much smaller as you want.

5. Two cups of water, as well as a trivet, should be added to the pot.

6. Place three ramekins on the trivet, accompanied by another three ramekins. Stack these in an overlapping fashion on top of the ramekins below, not directly onto the top of each other. Cook over low pressure for about 2 mins if you want runny yolks, three mins if you want rough yolks.

7. Speedy reduces pressure after the cooking period is over. Remove the lids and place the ramekins on a cooling rack for cooling. Serve right away.

NUTRITION: Calories: 155 kcal Fat: 11 g Protein: 10 g Carbs: 25 g

10. Cottage Pie with Cauliflower Mash

Ready in: 75 minutes

Servings: 10

Difficulty: Difficult

INGREDIENTS

- 10 oz chopped green beans

- 3 tbsp olive oil

- 1 tbsp oregano

- 2 lb beef

- Two minced garlic cloves

- One sliced onion

- 1 tsp salt

- Three chopped celery sticks

- 3 tbsp tomato paste

- ¼ cup vinegar

- 1 cup beef stock

- 2 tbsp thyme

Topping

- One pinch of paprika

- 1.6 lb chopped cauliflower

- ½ tsp salt

- 3 oz butter

- ¼ tsp pepper

- One pinch of dried oregano

- Three egg yolks

DIRECTIONS

1. Over higher heat, place a big saucepan.

2. Add the onion, oregano, garlic, olive oil, and celery to the pan & cook around 5 minutes, or until your onion is translucent.

3. Stir in the salt & beef as it browns.

4. Once the beef is browned, stir in tomato paste thoroughly.

5. Simmer uncovered around 20 mins till this liquid has reduced, then add both beef stock & vinegar.

6. Simmer for around 5 minutes with the thyme & green beans.

7. Remove the pan from the flame.

8. Fill the casserole dish halfway with some beef mixture, then set aside. The sauce is ready.

9. Preheat the oven to around 350 Fahrenheit.

10. Bring a big saucepan of water to a boil and add cauliflower.

11. Cook around 7 to 10 minutes, or until cauliflower is soft and drain.

12. Return your drained cauliflower with pepper, salt, and butter to the saucepan and cook for few minutes.

13. Blend the mixture in the blender with egg yolks.

14. In your casserole bowl, softly spoon the crushed cauliflower over the beef mixture.

15. Paprika & oregano can be sprinkled on top.

16. Bake the pie in preheated oven for 25 to 30 minutes

17. Serve right away, or chill & prepare for up to a week in the fridge.

NUTRITION: Calories: 420 kcal Fat: 36 g Protein: 18 g Carbs: 8 g

11. Tuna Stuffed Avocado

Ready in: 15 minutes

Servings: 2

Difficulty: Easy

INGREDIENTS

- 1 tsp lime juice

- 5 oz can tuna

- Two red onions, diced

- One avocado

- ¼ cup cilantro, diced

- 1 tsp mayo

- 2 tsp olive oil

- Salt to taste

- Lime for serving

- Black pepper to taste

DIRECTIONS

1. Scrape out most avocado, causing a small amount close to the skin to retain the avocado's form and mash the avocado.

2. Then, in a mixing bowl, combine the mashed avocado, olive oil, mayonnaise, salt, lime juice, and pepper.

3. Drain the tuna & add it to the avocado mix.

4. Then add the sliced cilantro & red onion, then whisk gently.

5. Sprinkle black pepper and salt.

6. Fill each avocado halves with the mixture and enjoy it.

NUTRITION: Calories: 407 kcal Fat: 5.1 g Protein: 19 g Carbs: 11 g

12. Foil – Packet Seafood with Beans and Kale

Ready in: 35 minutes

Servings: 4

Difficulty: Medium

INGREDIENTS

- 15 oz cherry Tomatoes

- 2 tbsp olive oil

- 15 oz beans

- ¼ cup wine

- ½ tsp red chili

- Two cloves chopped garlic

- ½ tsp oregano

- ½ loaf ciabatta

- Salt to taste

- One packet chopped kale

- Black pepper to taste

- Four halibut fillets

- 1 lb mussels

- 2 tbsp crushed parsley

DIRECTIONS

1. Preheat the grill to medium-high heat. On the work surface, set out four 12 x18" sheets of heavy-duty foil. In a big mixing cup, blend the peppers, oregano, beans, red pepper flakes, garlic, wine, olive oil, 3/4 teaspoon salt, & some grinds of pepper. Stir all together thoroughly.

2. Drizzle olive oil over the foil. Place kale into the middle of every sheet in an even layer. Place the halibut on top of, then season with salt & pepper. Place the mussels on the sheets and cover with the tomato mixture. Fold the sides to secure the foil by pulling the two small ends close and folding twice.

3. Grill the foil packages for about 10 minutes, or until this fish is baked through & the mussels have opened. Transfer to the baking sheet with caution. 1-2 mins per foot, grill your bread until finely charred. Season the side cuts with salt, then drizzle with olive oil. Cautiously remove each foil packet; remove any mussels that have not been opened. Offer with bread & a parsley garnish.

NUTRITION: Calories: 228 kcal Fat: 11.9 g Protein: 23.7 g Carbs: 8.9 g

13. Barramundi en Papillote

Ready in: 35 minutes

Servings: 5

Difficulty: Easy

INGREDIENTS

- One lemon juice

- 2 tbsp olive oil

- Two sliced capsicums (red and yellow)

- 200 g barramundi Fillets

- One chopped onion

- Two cloves chopped garlic

- 400 gm chopped cherry tomatoes

- 100 ml wine

- 2 tbsp chopped thyme

Fennel Salad

- Lemon to taste

- 2 Fennel Bulbs, cut into sliced

- 2 tbsp chopped parsley

- ¼ chopped Spanish onion

- 1 ½ tbsp olive oil

DIRECTIONS

1. Preheat the oven to almost 350 Fahrenheit. In the wide saucepan, heat the oil over medium to high heat, then add the onion, capsicum, and garlic, stirring regularly until soft. Simmer until the wine has been decreased by half, then add the saffron, thyme, & tomatoes, season to taste, & proceed to cook until the sauce has thickened (2-3 minutes). Thyme can be discarded.

2. Put four-wide sheets of baking sheet on the work surface, then uniformly spoon the capsicum mixture into the middle of each. Season to taste, then cover each part with a fish fillet,

drizzle with the oil & lemon juice, sprinkle with rind, then roll baking sheet over to shape parcels, dipping ends under it to seal. Switch to a baking sheet, then roast until the fish is just finished.

3. Meanwhile, to create the fennel salad, add the drained fennel with the remaining ingredients in a mixing bowl, season to taste, and toss to coat. Offer with the lemon wedges on top of the fish.

NUTRITION: Calories: 4212 kcal Fat: 18 g Protein: 2 g Carbs: 11 g

14. Provencal fish Stew

Ready in: 50 minutes

Servings: 4

Difficulty: Medium

INGREDIENTS

- 3 tbsp black olives

- 4 tbsp olive oil

- One crushed onion

- One chopped bulb fennel cored

- 2 tsp crushed thyme

- One chopped zucchini

- Salt to taste

- Two chopped garlic cloves

- 28 oz chopped tomatoes

- ½ cup dry wine

- 3 cups chicken soup

- 1 tsp saffron

- 1 ½ lb fish

- 8 oz potatoes

- One orange juice

- 3 tbsp fish basil leaves

DIRECTIONS

1. In a big Roasting pan or kettle, heat 2 tbsp olive oil over moderate heat. Sauté the fennel & onions for 5 minutes, or before they begin to become soft. Season with pepper and salt, then add the zucchini and garlic and roast for the next 5 minutes, or till all these vegetables are tender. Stir throughout white wine, wiping off any browned pieces from the base of the container.

2. Bring the tomatoes, pulp, broth, thyme, and saffron to a simmer; introduce the potatoes, cook for 10-12 mins, or soft.

1. Meanwhile, in a broad skillet on medium melt, heat the leftover 2 tbsp olive oil. Season your fish with pepper and salt,

then sear it on all sides for 5-7 minutes per hand until it's only barely grilled through. Take the fish from the pan & put it aside to cool slightly before cutting it into 1" pieces with a fork. Stir gently to mix them with the juice and orange zest, as well as the halved olives.

2. Ladle into the individual bowls and eat hot with the slivered basil over each piece. Place the slices of baguette mostly on the side or over the bowls with some rouille.

NUTRITION: Calories: 464.34 kcal Fat: 17.84 g Protein: 39.77 g Carbs: 34.64 g

Chapter 11: Snacks Recipes

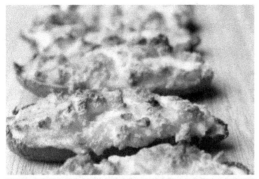

THE BEST
KETO SNACK
RECIPES

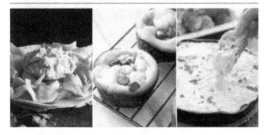

1. Parmesan – Roasted cauliflower

Ready in: 45 minutes

Servings: 6

Difficulty: Medium

INGREDIENTS

- 1 cup chopped cheese, gruyere

- One cauliflower, sliced

- Salt to taste

- 3 tbsp olive oil

- 1 cup chopped parmesan cheese

DIRECTIONS

1. Preheat the oven to approx. 350 Fahrenheit s.

2. Remove outer leaves from cauliflower & cut its head into the florets. Discard the stems. Place its florets on a sheet pan. Drizzle it with olive oil & sprinkle it generously with salt & pepper. Toss it well. Then bake for 30 min, tossing it once, till cauliflower is soft & starts to get browned. Sprinkle it with Parmesan & Gruyere, then bake for an additional 1-2 min, just till cheese melts. Season it to taste & serve warm.

NUTRITION: Calories: 247 kcal Fat: 18 g Protein: 6 g Carbs: 14 g

2. Rutabaga Fries

Ready in: 60 minutes

Servings: 3

Difficulty: Medium

INGREDIENTS

- 1 tsp chopped parsley

- Three rutabaga

- 3 cups water

- Salt to taste

- 2 tbsp olive oil

- 1 tsp chopped garlic

- Black pepper to taste

Toppings

- ¼ cup bacon bits

- ½ cup chopped cheese

DIRECTIONS

1. Peel the rutabaga & cut it into 1/4" thick pieces that resemble fries. Fry, if you desire more of the steak cut, also you may cut them thicker. Now to make the rutabagas easy to cut, place them in the microwave for about 30 secs / so to soften them.

2. Toss cut pieces of rutabaga into a bowl that has cold water with 1 tsp salt. Let it soak for 20 mins at least.

3. Preheat your oven to 400 Fahrenheit s.

4. Drain the water from the bowl. Now add olive oil, 1 tsp salt, garlic powder, pepper, & parsley. Toss it, make sure all the fries are finely coated.

5. Pour the seasoned fries on a baking sheet that would be lined with parchment paper. Spread it out evenly & bake in the oven for 30 mins. Toss the fries around & flip. Bring the oven to 425 Fahrenheit s & bake it for an additional 10 mins.

6. Serve & enjoy.

NUTRITION: Calories: 115 kcal Fat: 5 g Protein: 2 g Carbs: 12 g

3. Strawberry Crisp Recipe

Ready in: 45 minutes

Servings: 8

Difficulty: Medium

INGREDIENTS

Filling

- Five heaping cups of hulled and quartered fresh strawberries,

- 1 tsp vanilla extract

- 1/4 cup of granulated white sugar

- 3 Tbsps cornstarch

Topping

- 1 cup of all-purpose flour

- 3/4 cup of old fashioned oats

- 2/3 cup of packed brown sugar

- 1/2 tsp salt

- 2/3 cup of granulated white sugar

- 3/4 tsp cinnamon

- 1/2 cup of (1 stick) melted butter

DIRECTIONS

1. Preheat the oven to almost 350 Fahrenheit.

2. In a large mixing cup, combine the diced strawberries & sugar and whisk until the strawberries consume enough sugar. Stir in the vanilla extract & cornstarch until strawberries are fully covered. Pour this in the baking dish that has been packed.

3. Combine the rice, peas, salt, granulated sugar, brown sugar, and cinnamon in a different medium mixing cup. Stir throughout melted butter until it is uniformly spread and crumbly. Using a fork, uniformly spread this crumb mixture over the strawberries.

4. Bake 35 to 40 mins, or until the fruit is bubbly and the topping gets golden brown, in a preheated oven. Enable to cool for a few minutes before serving. Serve with a scoop of vanilla ice-cream on top when it's still soft.

NUTRITION: Calories: 387 Cal Fat: 12 g Protein: 3 g Carbs: 67 g

4. Cheesy Zucchini Casserole

Ready in: 45 minutes

Servings: 6

Difficulty: Medium

INGREDIENTS

- 2 to 3 zucchini, about 1/4-inch thick

- 1/4 tsp salt

- Three eggs

- 1/4 cup of grated parmesan cheese

- 3 to 4 garlic cloves, minced

- 1/3 cup of heavy cream

- 1 tsp dried basil

- 1/8 tsp ground nutmeg

- 1/4 tsp fresh ground pepper

- 1 1/2 cups divided shredded cheddar cheese

- 2 tbsps butter, sliced in 1/4-inch thick pieces

- Fresh parsley chopped for garnish

DIRECTIONS

1. Preheat the oven to almost 350 Fahrenheit.

2. Butter a 9" baking dish and put it aside.

3. Toss your sliced zucchini with the salt into a baking dish, then put aside.

4. Combine the nutmeg, heavy cream, garlic, parmesan cheese, eggs, basil, and ground pepper in a mixing dish.

5. Cover the zucchini with 1/2 cup sliced cheddar cheese.

6. Drizzle the ready cream sauce on the zucchini, then sprinkle the butter bits on top.

7. Bake for twenty minutes at 350 Fahrenheit.

8. Take these out of the oven, then top with the leftover cheese.

9. Bake for another 7 to 10 minutes, just until the zucchini is soft and bubbly.

10. Take these out of the oven & put them aside for 10 minutes.

11. Garnish with the parsley before cutting and serving.

NUTRITION: Calories: 256 Cal Fat: 22 g Protein: 13 g Carbs: 4 g

5. Pepperoni & Jalapeno Pizza

Ready in: 30 minutes

Servings: 8

Difficulty: Easy

INGREDIENTS

- 14 ounces whole peeled tomatoes

- 1 tsp oregano

- 1 tbsp Olive oil

- 1 tsp Dried basil

- 1/2 tsp Kosher Salt

- 1/4 tsp Ground black pepper

- 8 ounces shredded cheese

- One whole Pizza dough

- Pepperoni

- Chopped Jalapeno peppers

DIRECTIONS

1. Preheat the oven to almost 450 Fahrenheit.

2. Drain and puree canned tomatoes in the food processor.

3. Pulse together the salt, dried basil, oregano, olive oil, and pepper.

4. Layer the sauce thinly over the pizza dough, allowing a half-inch border for the crust.

5. Toss in the cheese, pepperoni, & jalapenos.

6. Bake for 8-10 mins, or until the cheese melts & the crust becomes golden brown. Take the baking sheet from the oven.

7. Cut into slices & serve.

NUTRITION: Calories: 294 Cal Fat: 4 g Protein: 10 g Carbs: 57 g

6. Easy Pizza Sauce

Ready in: 1-2 hours

Servings: 8

Difficulty: Easy

INGREDIENTS

- One can of tomato paste (6 ounces)

- 1 ½ cups of water

- ⅓ cup of extra virgin olive oil

- ½ tbsp basil

- Two cloves garlic, minced

- salt

- ground black pepper

- ½ tbsp oregano

- ½ tsp rosemary

DIRECTIONS

1. Combine the water, tomato paste, & olive oil in a mixing cup. Mix thoroughly. Garlic, oregano, salt & pepper to taste, basil, & rosemary are also good additions. Mix thoroughly and set aside for many hours to allow flavors to meld. There's no need to prepare it; just spread it on the dough.

NUTRITION: Calories: 104 Cal Fat: 9.5 g Protein: 1 g Carbs: 4.7 g

7. Peanut Butter Fat Bombs

Ready in: 1 hour 30 minutes

Servings: 1

Difficulty: Difficult

INGREDIENTS

Peanut Butter Fat Bombs

- 1/2 cup of coconut oil (melted)

- one tsp vanilla essence

  - 3/4 cup peanut butter

- 1/4 tsp salt

- 2 tsp liquid stevia

Chocolate Ganache

- Cocoa powder

- Coconut oil

- Liquid stevia

DIRECTIONS

1. Add the coconut oil, vanilla extract, spice, peanut butter, and liquid stevia in a mixing cup. Whisk until the paste is thick and creamy.

2. Use muffin paper-cups to fill a six-muffin tray. Fill each cup with around 3 tbsp of the peanut butter mixture.

3. Set aside for at least 1 hour or overnight in the refrigerator.

4. Mix some ganache components till it gets silky smooth as a peanut butter coating is chilling.

5. Top each fat bomb with around 1 tbsp of chocolate ganache.

6. Chill for almost 30 mins before serving in the refrigerator.

NUTRITION: Calories: 247 Cal Fat: 24.4 g Protein: 3.6 g Carbs: 3.3 g

8. Rosemary Roasted Rutabaga

Ready in: 45 minutes

Servings: 4

Difficulty: Medium

INGREDIENTS

- 1 tbsp butter

- 1 lb Rutabaga, sliced

- 1 tbsp crushed rosemary

- ¼ cup chopped onion

- 1 tbsp olive oil

- 1/8 tsp chili

- Salt to taste

DIRECTIONS

1. Firstly, preheat the oven to 400 Fahrenheit & place the rack in a middle position. Place a sheet pan with parchment paper.

2. Then toss cubed rutabaga with onion, rosemary, olive oil, pepper, salt, & spread it on the sheet pan in a flat layer. Bake for 20-30 mins or till your fork-tender.

3. Now heat a med-large frying pan over med heat. When it is hot, add some butter & swirl to coat your pan. Then fry this rutabaga till browned.

4. You can serve with grilled, roasted meats, or pan-seared, & a side salad here to minimize your extra carbs.

NUTRITION: Calories: 100 kcal Fat: 6.51 g Protein: 1.47 g Carbs: 10 g

9. Toum

Ready in: 30 minutes

Servings: 18

Difficulty: Easy

INGREDIENTS

- ½ cup lemon juice

- 1 cup chopped garlic

- 3 cups oil

- Salt to taste

DIRECTIONS

1. Firstly, slice the garlic cloves in half lengthwise & then you will remove any green sprouts.

2. Now transfer these sliced garlic cloves into a good food processor & add the salt to the garlic cloves. Process for 1 min till the garlic will turn finely minced. Make sure to scrape down these sides of your food processor afterward.

3. When the food processor is running, you slowly pour 1-2 tbsps of oil, and then you will stop it & scrape down your bowl. Continue it & add another tbsp or two till the garlic starts in a creamy texture.

4. Once the garlic looks creamy by the few tbsps of oil, then increase your speed of pouring the oil & alternate with the half cup of lemon juice till all the lemon juice & oil is incorporated. This will have taken about 15 mins to complete.

5. Now transfer this sauce into a glass container & then cover it with a paper towel in your fridge overnight.

NUTRITION: Calories: 343 kcal Fat: 37 g Protein: 1 g Carbs: 3 g

10. Turnip Slaw

Ready in: 20 minutes

Servings: 4

Difficulty: Easy

INGREDIENTS

- 4 cups chopped turnips

- ¼ cup sliced red chili

- Salt to taste

- 1 tbsp vinegar

- ¼ cup melt mayonnaise

- 2 tbsp sugar

- Black pepper to taste

DIRECTIONS

1. In the bowl, mix all the ingredients except turnips. Now pour over the turnips & toss it well to coat. Then refrigerate for several hrs for its flavors to blend.

NUTRITION: Calories: 113 kcal Fat: 4 g Protein: 2 g Carbs: 18 g

11. Carrot and Red Cabbage slaw with Turnips and Dressing

Ready in: 40 minutes

Servings: 5

Difficulty: Medium

INGREDIENTS

- ½ cup crushed cilantro

- 4 cups chopped Turnips

- ½ chopped cabbage

- Two chopped carrot

- 3 Choy leaves

Slaw Dressing

- 1 tbsp syrup

- ¼ cup olive oil

- One bulb chopped garlic

- One lemon Juice

- 1 tbsp soy sauce

DIRECTIONS

1. Shred the turnips & carrots, then add to a large bowl. You can shred them using a large box grater and shred them in a food processor with a shredding blade.

2. After it, make thin slices of red cabbage & bok choy, then add them to a larger bowl. Now add turnips, cabbage, carrots, cilantro, & bok choy to bowl & toss well.

3. In the small bowl, mix all the dressing ingredients.

4. Then pour dressings over vegetables & herbs in a large bowl & mix well

NUTRITION: Calories: 185 kcal Fat: 11 g Protein: 3 g Carbs: 20 g

12. Grilled Fresh onions

Ready in: 25 minutes

Servings: 5

Difficulty: Easy

INGREDIENTS

- Black pepper to taste

- 1 lb chopped onion

- 2 tbsp lemon juice

- 2 tbsp olive oil

- Salt to taste

DIRECTIONS

1. Preheat the oven to 400 Fahrenheit. Now split those onions in lengthwise half & put them on a baking dish.

2. Drizzle the lemon juice & oil on top, then season it using pepper & salt to taste. Then in the oven, roast it for about 20 mins till the onion is tender & finely browned.

3. If you are about to cook onions on the grill, mix lemon juice & oil in a small bowl. Cut onions in lengthwise half & brush them using oil/lemon mix. Season using salt & pepper to taste.

4. Grill it for 10-15 mins (depends on its size) & turn after every few min.

5. Serve it right after it gets off from grill / at room temp & drizzle with remaining lemon juice & oil right before serving.

NUTRITION: Calories: 135 kcal Fat: 10 g Protein: 1 g Carbs: 9 g

13. Zucchini Fries with Spicy Tomato Mayo

Ready in: 25 minutes

Servings: 4

Difficulty: Easy

INGREDIENTS

- 3 tbsp olive oil

- 2 lb Zucchini

- Two eggs

- 1 tsp onion paste

- 4 oz Almond flour

- Black pepper to taste

Spicy tomato Mayo

- Black pepper to taste

- 1 cup Mayonnaise

- ½ tsp chili

- 1 tsp chopped tomato

- Salt to taste

DIRECTIONS

1. Mix the ingredients for tomato mayo & refrigerate.

2. To 400 Fahrenheit, preheat the oven. Line the baking sheet using parchment paper.

3. In a bowl, crack the eggs & whisk till smooth.

4. Mix the almond flour, spices & parmesan cheese in the other bowl.

5. Cut zucchini into sticks & remove seeds.

6. Dredge zucchini sticks in almond flour mixt till they're completely covered. Then dip them in egg batter & then again in the almond flour mix.

7. Place zucchini sticks on a baking sheet & drizzle on olive oil. Bake it in the oven for almost 20-25 mins / till fries have browned finely. Serve it along with spicy tomato mayo.

NUTRITION: Calories: 843 kcal Fat: 78 g Protein: 24 g Carbs: 8 g

14. Caramelized Endives with Apples

Ready in: 40 minutes

Servings: 4

Difficulty: Medium

INGREDIENTS

- ½ cup water

- One sliced smith apple

- Salt to taste

- 1 tbsp butter

- 4 Belgian, sliced

- 1 tbsp cooking oil

DIRECTIONS

1. Carefully tuck the six apple slices b/w leaves in each half of the endive. Now in a large pan, melt butter in oil on high heat. Add endives, cut its sides down, & cook on moderate heat till finely browned, almost for 6 min. Now carefully turn those endives. Season it using salt & pepper, then add water to the pan. Cover & simmer on low heat till endives are tender, for 12-15 mins. Now uncover & cook till the liquid has evaporated & serve hot.

NUTRITION: Calories: 290 kcal Fat: 29 g Protein: 3 g Carbs: 1 g

15. Caramelized Endives with Creamy Pumpkin Pasta

Ready in: 35 minutes

Servings: 1

Difficulty: Medium

INGREDIENTS

- 1 tbsp olive oil

- Six chopped endives

- Three chopped shallots

- 1 cup orange juice

- 1 tbsp soy sauce

- ½ tsp basil

- 1 tbsp maple syrup

- Black pepper to taste

- ½ tbsp almonds powder

- ½ tsp nutmeg

- Cheese

Pumpkin pasta

- 1 ½ vegetable soup

- 7 oz spaghetti

- 1 cup coconut milk

- ½ cup pumpkin

- One bulb garlic paste

- Salt to taste

- ¼ tsp chili

DIRECTIONS

Caramelized endives

1. In a pan, heat the oil on med heat, add shallots, & cook for 3-5 mins /until they start to brown.

2. Now rinse endives, remove their outer leaves & trim from the bottom. Add it to the pan & brown for 1-2 mins, flip them once.

3. Pour it in orange juice, soy sauce, maple syrup, nutmeg & black pepper. Turn heat on high & cover. Cook it for at least 30 mins.

4. Once the endives are soft & may be pierced easily with a knife, now uncover & let the rest of the liquid evaporate & when no liquid stands, continue the cooking till they caramelize, turn them regularly to brown them evenly.

5. Serve with roasted almonds, pumpkin pasta, & crumbled cheese.

Pot pumpkin pasta

1. In the large saucepan, mix pumpkin puree, garlic, chili, coconut milk, water, & salt. Now simmer on med heat. Then add spaghetti & cook for 8-9 mins (or less, depends upon which pasta you have), regularly mixing to prevent it from sticking. Watch it carefully as the liquid will rise quickly. Taste & adjust the seasonings if needed.

NUTRITION: Calories: 305 kcal Fat: 8.3 g Protein: 10.3 g Carbs: 50 g

Chapter 12: Soup Recipes

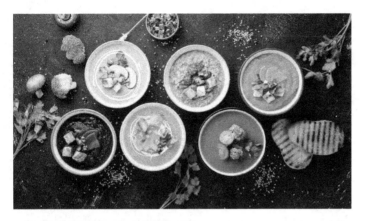

1. Chorizo Tortilla Soup

Ready in: 50 minutes

Servings: 20

Difficulty: Medium

INGREDIENTS

- 1 cup crushed onion

- 12 oz Spanish

- 2 tbsp olive oil

- 28 oz chopped tomatoes

- 4 cups chicken soup

- Salt to taste

- 2 tsp garlic paste

- 15 oz beans

- 2 cups tomatoes ketchup

- Black pepper to taste

DIRECTIONS

1. In oil, mix onion for 4 to 6 minutes, mix garlic for 60 seconds, and then on the other pan, cook sausage in oil for 4 min till brown color.

2. Mix chicken broth, salt, tomatoes, and potatoes and boil them for 6 minutes, then mix beans in it and stir for 20 to 21 minutes. In other pans, fry tortilla pieces for 60 seconds, spread the salt, flavor the soup with salt and pepper, and serve it with tortilla strips.

NUTRITION: Calories: 325.7 kcal Fat: 19.6 g Protein: 15 g Carbs: 21.3 g

2. Stew Like Soup

Ready in: 35 minutes

Servings: 4

Difficulty: Easy

INGREDIENTS

- 2 tbsp olive oil

- 1 lb chicken

- Black pepper to taste

- Three cloves chopped garlic

- One crushed onion

- One red chili

- Salt to taste

- Six chopped potatoes

- 15 oz red kidney beans

- 15 oz chopped potatoes, fire-roasted

- 2 tsp sauce

- 1 cup corn tortilla chips

- ¼ cup chicken stock

- ¾ lb Chorizo Sausage

- 2 cup smoked cheddar

- Crushed cilantro

- Crushed scallions

- Chopped thyme

DIRECTIONS

1. Mix chicken with salt and pepper, combine chicken and oil in a pan till brown color, then put chorizo and garlic and bake it for 4 minutes.

2. Now mix potatoes, peppers, and onions.

3. Then cook with hot sauce, tomatoes, kidney beans for 4 to 6 minutes.

4. Mix chicken broth and boil it for 10 minutes.

5. Serve it with tortillas and cheese, with garnishing of scallions and herbs.

NUTRITION: Calories: 774 kcal Fat: 42.9 g Protein: 36.9 g Carbs: 61.7 g

3. Rosemary Lamb Stew

Ready in: 125 minutes

Servings: 5

Difficulty: Difficult

INGREDIENTS

- Six chopped mushroom

- ½ lb lamb meat

- ½ sliced of onion

- One chopped potato

- ¼ cup flour

- 2 tbsp olive oil

- 3 cup chicken soup

- Two stalks crushed celery

- 2 tbsp chopped rosemary

- ½ tsp chopped thyme

- ¼ tsp sage

- ½ tsp paprika

- ¼ tsp oregano

- Salt to taste

- 2 tsp wine

- Black pepper to taste

- ½ tsp sauce

DIRECTIONS

1. In oil, cook onion, celery, and mushroom and put on the plate.

2. Now mix the meat in oil and cook from all sides till brown color.

3. Spread the paprika and then flour and cook till flour browned.

4. Now combine broth and stir, finally combine all the meat ingredients and boil it for 60 minutes.

NUTRITION: Calories: 217 kcal Fat: 8.7 g Protein: 17.2 g Carbs: 16.8 g

4. Bacon Cauliflower Chowder

Ready in: 35 minutes

Servings: 5

Difficulty: Medium

INGREDIENTS

- 1 cup milk

- Four chopped bacon

- Two crushed carrot

- One crushed onion

- Salt to taste

- Two stalks crushed celery

- 2 tbsp flour

- Black pepper to taste

- ¼ cup vegetable soup

- Two cloves chopped garlic

- Two chopped thyme

DIRECTIONS

1. In a pan, cook bacon till they become crispy; in another pan, mix celery, onions, and carrot with salt and pepper and cook it for 6 minutes.

2. Now cook garlic for 60 seconds and then add flour, thyme, and cauliflower and cook it for 120 seconds.

3. Add broth and milk and simmer till tender the cauliflower for 16 to 20 minutes.

4. Finally, flavor it and garnish it with salt, pepper, and bacon.

NUTRITION: Calories: 249 kcal Fat: 5 g Protein: 10 g Carbs: 207 g

5. Creamy Cauliflower and Potato Soup with Bacon

Ready in: 35 minutes

Servings: 4

Difficulty: Medium

INGREDIENTS

- 6 cup cream

- 1 tbsp olive oil

- 250 g crushed bacon

- Two chopped leeks

- Three cloves chopped garlic

- ¼ cauliflower, cut into sliced

- Bread

- 500 g chopped potatoes

DIRECTIONS

1. Cook bacon in heated oil for 180 seconds.

2. Mix garlic in oil, put in the pan, a cook for 4 to 6 minutes.

3. Mix stock, potato, and boil after adding cauliflower. Boil it for 30 minutes till all the vegetables become soft.

4. Mix soup in sets till it smooth and mix in the cream and heat it and then pour it into the pot spread pepper on it and top with bacon and serve it and enjoy it.

NUTRITION: Calories: 1270 kcal Fat: 10.7 g Protein: 25 g Carbs: 26.4 g

6. Chicken and Kale Soup

Ready in: 45 minutes

Servings: 6

Difficulty: Medium

INGREDIENTS

- Two chopped potatoes

- 1 tbsp olive oil

- 1 tbsp chopped garlic

- Two chopped thyme

- 1 ½ cups crushed onion

- 15 oz North beans

- 12 oz boneless chicken

- 6 cups chicken soup

- 3 cups crushed kale

- Salt to taste

- 2 tbsp lemon juice

- Black pepper to taste

DIRECTIONS

1. Mix onion in heated oil for 4 to 6 minutes, put garlic in it, and then combine beans, salt broth, pepper, potatoes, and thyme.

2. Boil the mixture on medium to high flame.

3. Add chicken in the form of pieces, mix kale in soup, and bake it till kale is softened.

4. Finally, mix it with shredded chicken and lemon juice. Serve it and enjoy it.

NUTRITION: Calories: 271 kcal Fat: 5.1 g Protein: 25.8 g Carbs: 30.4 g

7. Cheeseburger Soup

Ready in: 45 minutes

Servings: 12

Difficulty: Medium

INGREDIENTS

- 3 cup chicken stock

- ½ lb beef

- ¾ cup grated carrot

- ¾ cup diced onion

- ¾ cup chopped celery

- 1 tsp parsley, dried

- 1 tsp basil, dried

- 4 tbsp butter

- 4 cup chopped potatoes

- ¼ cup all-purpose flour

- ¾ tsp salt

- 2 cups processed cheese

- ½ tsp black pepper

- 1 ½ cup milk

- ¼ cup sour cream

DIRECTIONS

1. Sauté the ground beef by browning it in the saucepan. And then drain it before setting it aside.

2. Then add some butter, shredded carrot, basil, onion, parsley flakes, and celery in the same pan and cook until they are done.

3. Add beef, potatoes, and broth and boil it. Cook it until the potatoes become tender.

4. Melt butter and then mix in the flour in the small skillet. Stir until it gets bubbly. Transfer it into a soup and boil it. Cook it for 3 minutes while keep stirring it.

5. Add cheese, salt, milk, and pepper, and cook until the cheese melts. Stop heating and mix it in sour cream.

6. Serve and enjoy it.

NUTRITION: Calories: 258 kcal Fat: 14 g Protein: 15 g Carbs: 19 g

8. Harvest Pork Stew

Ready in: 25 minutes

Servings: 6

Difficulty: Easy

INGREDIENTS

- 1 cup cider vinegar

- 2 lb pork tenderloin

- 10 oz butternut squash

- 1 cup chopped carrot

- Three garlic cloves

- One apple, honey crisp

- ½ cup chopped onion

- One smith apple

- 3 cups chicken stock

- 1 tsp thyme, dried

- 1 tsp paprika

- ¼ tsp chili powder

- 2 tbsp tapioca pearls

- 4 tbsp tomato paste

- ½ tsp salt

- ½ tsp sage, dried

DIRECTIONS

1. Combine all the items in a cooker and stir well.

2. Cover the cooker and let it cook for 5 hours at high flame.

3. Serve and enjoy it.

NUTRITION: Calories: 312.86 kcal Fat: 6.5 g Protein: 35.5 g Carbs: 30 g

9. Lasagna Soup

Ready in: 50 minutes

Servings: 6

Difficulty: Medium

INGREDIENTS

- ½ tsp thyme, dried

- 2 tbsp olive oil

- One chopped onion

- 1 lb ground beef

- Five minced garlic cloves

- 14.5 oz chopped tomatoes

- 4 ½ cup chicken stock

- 14.5 oz mashed tomatoes

- One ¾ tsp basil, dried

- 2 ½ tbsp tomato paste

- ¾ tsp oregano, dried

- Black pepper to taste

- ½ tsp rosemary, dried

- 6 oz lasagna noodles

- Salt to taste

- ½ cup grated parmesan

- 8 oz ricotta cheese

- One ¼ cup grated mozzarella cheese

- 2 tbsp diced parsley

DIRECTIONS

1. Heat the olive oil and cook the beef pieces, relished with pepper and salt, in the pot. Stir the beef periodically until it gets browned. After draining the fat, set the beef aside.

2. Now sauté the chopped onions for almost 4 minutes inside the olive oil until they get soft, and then add some garlic and heat it for 1 minute.

3. . Add diced and crushed tomatoes, basil, chicken broth, oregano, tomato paste, thyme, browned beef, and rosemary.

4. Oil it and then reduce the flame to medium and keep it simmer and cover for almost 23 minutes.

5. According to the instructions listed on the package, prepare the lasagna noodles.

6. Mix ricotta, mozzarella, and parmesan in a mixing bowl using a fork.

7. With parsley, mix the cooked pasta while stirring it into a soup. Thin the soup with broth if it is required.

8. Pour the soup into the bowl, add few scoops of cheese, and then sprinkle the soup with finely chopped parsley.

NUTRITION: Calories: 546 cal Fat: 26 g Protein: 38 g Carbs: 41 g

10. Beef Pumpkin Stew

Ready in: 250 minutes

Servings: 8

Difficulty: Medium

INGREDIENTS

- 1 tbsp Worcestershire sauce

- 3 lb beef

- 3 tbsp butter

- ½ cup all-purpose flour

- 1 cup diced onion

- 4 cups beef broth

- One minced garlic clove

- 3 cups pumpkin puree

- 3 lb chopped potatoes

- 1 tbsp salt

- Three sprigs of thyme

- 1 tsp black pepper

- 1 lb chopped carrot

DIRECTIONS

1. Cut beef into pieces and then cover all sides with flour.

2. Melt butter in a wide soup pot. Subject beef pieces to the flame until they all turn brown. Sauté onion and garlic into the pot for a short period while keep stirring for 2 minutes.

3. Add the brown beef pieces back into the pot and add pumpkin puree and beef stock, pepper, Worcestershire sauce, salt. Subject the pot to the flame until the ingredients are about to get a boil. Once the boiling state is achieved, mitigate the flame intensity to medium and let it simmer for 4 hours.

4. Add Carrots, thyme sprigs, and potatoes into the pot and keep the flame to. It is important to cook for 45 more minutes and add salt to impart taste to the meal. Serve and enjoy the meal.

NUTRITION: Calories: 650 cal Fat: 31 g Protein: 44 g Carbs: 48 g

11. Creamy Roasted Red Pepper Tomato Soup

Ready in: 30 minutes

Servings: 1

Difficulty: Easy

INGREDIENTS

- Two red bell peppers

- 6 oz tomato paste

- 28 oz mashed potatoes

- 1 cup water

- 14 oz coconut milk

- ½ tsp salt

- 1 ½ tbsps dills, dried

- 1 tsp basil, dried

- 1 tbsp garlic powder

- 3 ½ tbsp coconut sugar

- ½ tsp black pepper

- One pinch of red pepper flakes

For Serving

- Croutons

- Dill

- Sliced Tomatoes

- Crispy chickpeas, baked

- Coconut milk

DIRECTIONS

1. Roast red peppers in a 500 Fahrenheit oven until tender.

2. Wrap and steam for a few minutes. Meanwhile, add other soup ingredients to the pot and boil them. Unwrap and cool red peppers and remove outer skin seeds and also stems. Add them to the soup.

3. Transfer to the blender to blend the soup. Then transfer back to the pot and boil over low heat. Adjust seasonings as needed.

4. Cook it on low flame for at least 10 minutes. Serve it with croutons or dill. Enjoy.

NUTRITION: Calories: 161 kcal Fat: 0.4 g Protein: 7.1 g Carbs: 35.5 g

12. Broccoli Soup

Ready in: 40 minutes

Servings: 4

Difficulty: Medium

INGREDIENTS

- ½ cup cream

- 4 tbsp butter

- Pepper to taste

- One diced onion

- 1 ½ lb broccoli

- One sliced carrot

- Salt to taste

- 4 cups chicken stock

- 3 tbsp all-purpose flour

- Croutons

DIRECTIONS

1. Add broccoli, carrot, onion, salt, and pepper into butter and sauté until onion is soft.

2. Add flour and cook for a minute.

3. Add broth and boil. Cook until broccoli is soft. Add cream.

4. Blend the soup.

5. Add salt and pepper. Serve with Croutons. Enjoy.

NUTRITION: Calories: 207 kcal Fat: 12.4 g Protein: 9.2 g Carbs: 17 g

13. Creamy Asparagus Soup

Ready in: 45 minutes

Servings: 5

Difficulty: Medium

INGREDIENTS

- 1 tbsp vermouth, dry

- 2 lb asparagus

- 1 tsp garlic, smashed

- One diced onion

- 3 tbsp butter

- 1 cup water

- 4 cups broth

- 1 tsp salt

- Two thyme sprigs

- ¼ cup parsley, diced

- One bay leaf

- ¼ cup sour cream

- 1 tsp lemon juice

- ½ tsp black pepper

DIRECTIONS

1. In melted butter, mix onion and cook it for 4 minutes; cook it for 1 minute after adding garlic.

2. Now combine asparagus in the onion, and after that, add salt and pepper and cook for 6 minutes.

3. Mix bay leaf, water, broth with thyme sprigs, boil it and finally mix it with parsley.

4. Blanch asparagus tips and cook it for 5 minutes. Now blend the soup in a blender and mix it with cream and lemon juice.

Combine vermouth with it also. Serve with salt and pepper to taste.

NUTRITION: Calories: 196 kcal Fat: 13.4 g Protein: 6.6 g Carbs: 14.1 g

14. Chicken Avocado Lime Soup

Ready in: 25 minutes

Servings: 6

Difficulty: Easy

INGREDIENTS

- 1 tbsp olive oil

- Two smashed jalapenos

- 1 cup green onions, diced

- Two smashed garlic cloves

- 1 ½ cups of water

- 14.5 oz chicken stock

- Pepper to taste

- 2 ½ chicken breasts

- ½ tsp oregano

- Three sliced tomatoes

- ¼ tsp coriander

- Salt to taste

- Four diced radishes

- 3 tbsps lime juice

- 1/3 cup cilantro, diced

- Three sliced avocados

DIRECTIONS

1. In olive oil, cook green onions and jalapeno for 120 seconds.

2. Mix garlic and boil it for 1 minute.

3. Add chicken broth, chicken breast, salt, pepper, water, cumin, coriander, and oregano and boil it for `14 to 15 minutes. Remove the chicken and turn the heat down to medium-low.

4. Add the radishes.

5. Combine shredded chicken with cilantro and lime juice.

6. Mix avocados, also mix sour cream, crushed tortilla chips, cheese, and serve.

NUTRITION: Calories: 241 kcal Fat: 2 g Protein: 10 g Carbs: 12 g

15. Greek Lemon Chicken Soup

Ready in: 30 minutes

Servings: 8

Difficulty: Easy

INGREDIENTS

- ½ tsp red pepper, minced

- 10 cups chicken stock

- 3 tbsp olive oil

- Six smashed garlic

- One diced onion

- Two chicken breasts

- One lemon, zested

- 1 cup couscous

- 2 oz shredded cheese, feta

- Salt to taste

- 1/3 cup chive, diced

- Pepper to taste

DIRECTIONS

1. Cook garlic and onion in oil for 4 to 5 minutes.

2. Mix red pepper, chicken broth, lemon zest, and chicken breast and boil it for 6 to 7 minutes.

3. Add 1 Tsp salt and black pepper and boil for 6 minutes. With fork tong the chicken and mix it with chopped chive and feta cheese.

4. Serve and enjoy with salt and pepper to taste.

5. Using tongs, remove the two chicken breasts from the pot. Use a fork and tongs to shred the chicken.

6. Then place it back in the pot. Stir in the crumbled feta cheese and chopped chive.

7. Taste and salt and pepper as needed. Serve warm.

NUTRITION: Calories: 214 kcal Fat: 8 g Protein: 11 g Carbs: 23 g

16. Cream of Zucchini Soup

Ready in: 25 minutes

Servings: 4

Difficulty: Easy

INGREDIENTS

- Shredded cheese, parmesan

- ½ diced onion

- Three chopped zucchini

- Two minced garlic cloves

- 32 oz broth

- Salt to taste

- 2 tbsp sour cream

- Pepper to taste

DIRECTIONS

1. Boil the chicken broth with zucchini, onion, and garlic for 19 to 20 minutes.

2. Now blend it in a blender and mix it with cream and blend it till it becomes smooth.

3. Serve and enjoy it with salt and pepper to taste.

NUTRITION: Calories: 60 kcal Fat: 1 g Protein: 3 g Carbs: 10 g

Chapter 13: Salad Recipes

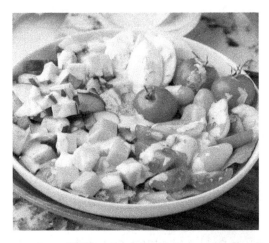

1. Cauliflower Potato Salad

Ready in: 35 minutes

Servings: 5

Difficulty: Easy

INGREDIENTS

- One tbsp of Dijon powder

- One cauliflower

- ½ tsp of paprika

- Two half-boiled eggs

- One tbsp vinegar

- Half tsp sea salt

- 1/3rd cup of chopped onion

- ¼ tsp of black pepper

- 2/3 cup of mayonnaise

- Chines for garnishing

DIRECTIONS

1. Take water in a pot and boil cauliflower till it is tendered. Add one tbsp of salt.

2. Mix the mayonnaise, vinegar, garlic powder, sea salt, pepper, and Dijon mustard till a smooth texture is obtained.

3. Add cauliflower, celery, eggs, and onion.

4. Stir continuously.

5. Garnish with chives.

6. Serve and enjoy.

NUTRITION: Calories: 94.3 Cal Fat: 7.4 g Protein: 3.1 g Carbs: 4 g

2. Steak Avocado Salad

Ready in: 30 minutes

Servings: 4

Difficulty: Easy

INGREDIENTS

- 2 cups of cherry tomatoes

- 460 g steak piece

- 2 tbsp oil

- Salt and pepper

- Two chopped hearts romaine

- Two diced avocados

- Three boiled eggs

- 3 tbsp Caesar dressing

DIRECTIONS

1. Season the steak with sea salt and pepper and rub it on the surface.

2. Take a pan and heat oil in it over medium flame.

3. Fry steak in it for 2-3 minutes from both sides properly.

4. Keep the steak on a separate plate for 10-15 minutes.

5. Makes the slices of steak.

6. Take a large bowl and mix all the ingredients.

7. Toss/mix until all the ingredients are well mixed.

8. Serve and enjoy.

NUTRITION: Calories: 577 cal Fat: 44 g Protein: 32 g Carbs: 15 g

3. Strawberry Cheesecake Salad

Ready in: 15 minutes

Servings: 8

Difficulty: Easy

INGREDIENTS

- Three sliced bananas

- 2 cup of cheesecake

- Three containers of strawberry yogurt

- 12 oz of whipped topping

- 1 lb sliced strawberries

- 3 cups of marshmallows

DIRECTIONS

1. Take a large bowl and whip the yogurt.

2. Place the bowl in the refrigerator.

3. Take the bowl out just before serving and add mix all the ingredients together.

4. Serve and enjoy.

NUTRITION: Calories: 459 cal Fat: 5 g Protein: 7 g Carbs: 25 g

4. Broccoli Cauliflower Salad

Ready in: 20 minutes

Servings: 6

Difficulty: Easy

INGREDIENTS

- 1/3 cup of raisins

- 3 cups cauliflower

- ½ red chopped onion

- 3 cups broccoli

- 1 cup grated cheddar

- ½ pack chopped bacon

- ¼ cup of sunflower seeds

- 1/3 cup of sugar

- 1 cup of mayonnaise

- ¼ cup white vinegar

DIRECTIONS

1. Take a pot and cook the bacon pieces. Keep aside to cool.

2. Take all the ingredients in a large bowl and mix well.

3. Serve and enjoy.

NUTRITION: Calories: 467 cal Fat: 38 g Protein: 8 g Carbs: 24 g

5. Monster Wedge Salad

Ready in: 35 minutes

Servings: 5

Difficulty: Easy

INGREDIENTS

Dressing

- ¼ cup Greek yogurt

- 1 tbsp of mayonnaise

- Salt & pepper

- 3 tbsp of sour cream

- 3 tbsp of milk

- ¼ cup cheese crumbles

- Worcestershire

- 2 tsp balsamic vinegar

Salad

- Chives

- Iceberg lettuce

- Four boiled eggs

- 1/3 cup of crumbled bacon

- Ten sliced grape tomatoes

DIRECTIONS

1. Take all the dressing ingredients in a large bowl and whisk well. Keep aside.

2. Take salad ingredients in a bowl and drizzle the dressing.

3. Top it with chives, blue cheese, tomatoes, and eggs.

4. Serve and enjoy.

NUTRITION: Calories: 201 cal Fat: 13 g Protein: 11 g Carbs: 8 g

6. Israeli salad

Ready in: 15 minutes

Servings: 8

Difficulty: Easy

INGREDIENTS

- Salt to taste

- 1 lb diced Persian cucumbers

- 3 tbsp lemon juice

- 1/3 cup of minced onion

- 1 lb diced tomatoes

- ½ cup minced parsley

- Black pepper to taste

DIRECTIONS

1. Cut all the vegetables into small sizes.

2. Take a large mixing bowl and mix all the ingredients well.

3. Add lemon juice.

4. Serve and enjoy.

NUTRITION: Calories: 70 cal Fat: 5 g Protein: 1 g Carbs: 5 g

7. Coastal Cobb Salad

Ready in: 15 minutes

Servings: 8

Difficulty: Easy

INGREDIENTS

- 2 cups of diced cucumbers

- Six cups of water

- ½ cup of sour cream

- 1 ½ peeled raw shrimp

- 6 tbsp of olive oil

- 1 tbsp of wine vinegar

- ¼ cup of buttermilk

- ¼ tsp of salt

- ½ tsp of black pepper

- Two chopped romaine lettuce

- 1 ounce of blue cheese

- 1 pt. quartered tomatoes

- 2 cups of shredded cabbage

- Two sliced carrots

- ½ cup of olives

- Eight boiled eggs

- ¼ cup of parsley leaves

DIRECTIONS

1. Boil water in a pot. And fill a separate bowl with ice.

2. Cook shrimp in boiling water. Drain and transfer in the ice bowl.

3. Mix well the olive, cream, buttermilk, vinegar, salt & pepper in a large bowl. Add blue cheese.

4. Make a layer of vegetables and put the dressing on the top. Place cooked shrimp in the middle and place olives & eggs around. Garnish with parsley.

5. Serve and enjoy.

NUTRITION: Calories: 548 cal Fat: 36 g Protein: 37.7 g Carbs: 17.7 g

8. Green Bean, Onion, Basil, and Tomato Salad

Ready in: 1 hour 15 minutes

Servings: 6

Difficulty: moderate

INGREDIENTS

- ½ sliced red onion

- 1/3 cup of snipped basil

- 2 tbsp of dried tomatoes

- 3 tbsp of red wine vinegar

- 1 tbsp olive oil

- ¼ tsp of pepper

- Two garlic cloves

- 12 oz green beans

- 8 oz tomatoes

- 8 oz red and yellow cherry

DIRECTIONS

1. Take a small bowl and stir together the basil, vinegar, tomatoes, olive oil, salt, garlic, and pepper.

2. Cook the green beans in a saucepan in salted water for 8-10 minutes. Drain and rinse well.

3. Take a large separate bowl and mix all the ingredients.

4. Serve and enjoy.

NUTRITION: Calories: 53 cal Fat: 2.5 g Protein: 1.7 g Carbs: 7.6 g

9. Shrimp and Cauliflower

Ready in 30 minutes

Servings: 6

Difficulty: Easy

INGREDIENTS

- ¼ cup of olive oil

- One cauliflower

- 2 tbsp of olive oil

- 1lb raw shrimp

- Two cucumbers

- ¼ cup lemon juice

- 3 tbsp chopped dill

- Salt to taste

- 2 tbsp lemon zest

- Black pepper to taste

DIRECTIONS

1. Cut the shrimp and season with olive oil, salt, and pepper.

2. Put it in the oven for 5-10 minutes at 350 Fahrenheit.

3. Cut and oven the cauliflower for 3-5 minutes.

4. Cool shrimp and cauliflower.

5. Cut other vegetables.

6. Take a large bowl and mix all the ingredients.

7. Add lemon juice and olive oil.

8. Toss well.

9. Serve and enjoy.

NUTRITION: Calories: 700 cal Fat: 70 g Protein: 67 g Carbs: 29 g

10. Caprese Zucchini Pasta

Ready in: 25 minutes

Servings: 4

Difficulty: Easy

INGREDIENTS

- 8 oz of fresh mozzarella

- 3 tbsp olive oil

- 12 oz tomatoes

- 2 lb of zucchini

- Two garlic cloves

- ½ cup basil leaves

- 2tbsp of capers

- ¼ cup almonds

DIRECTIONS

1. Take a large skillet and heat oil in it.

2. Cook zucchini for 1-2 minutes.

3. Transfer it to a large bowl.

4. Add mozzarella, garlic, tomatoes, basil, and salt.

5. Toss well.

6. Top with salted almonds.

7. Serve and enjoy.

NUTRITION: Calories: 166 cal Fat: 4 g Protein: 7 g Carbs: 4 g

11. Chimichurri Chicken Avocado Salad

Ready in: 20 minutes

Servings: 4

Difficulty: Easy

INGREDIENTS

- Two sliced avocadoes

- One batch chimichurri

- 1 tsp olive oil

- Four chicken thigh fillets

- 5 cups dried lettuce leaves

- ½ sliced red onion

- Three sliced tomatoes

- Parsley for garnishing

DIRECTIONS

1. Take chimichurri in a bowl and add 4tbsp of olive oil. Keep it to marinate for 15-20 minutes in the refrigerator.

2. Take a grill or skillet and heat oil in it over medium heat.

3. Grill the chicken fillets in a skillet from each side.

4. Make slices of chicken.

5. Cut the other vegetables.

6. Take a large bowl and mix all the ingredients.

7. Serve and enjoy.

NUTRITION: Calories: 449 cal Fat: 34 g Protein: 22 g Carbs: 15 g

12. Romaine Salad with Cheese and Bacon

Ready in: 30 minutes

Servings: 8

Difficulty: Easy

INGREDIENTS

- 1 cup of shredded mozzarella cheese

- 8 cups of lettuce

- 1 cup of drained pimientos

- ½ cup of parmesan cheese

- ½ cup of olive oil

- Ten crumbled bacon strips

- ¼ cup of cider vinegar

- Six sliced green onions

DIRECTIONS

1. Take a large bowl and mix onions, lettuce, cheese, bacon, and pimientos.

2. Take a separate bowl and whisk together the oil, cider, garlic powder, sugar, salt & pepper.

3. Pour it over the salad.

4. Toss well.

5. Garnish with croutons.

6. Serve and enjoy.

NUTRITION: Calories: 275 cal Fat: 21 g Protein: 10 g Carbs: 6 g

13. Tomato Mozzarella Salad

Ready in 20 minutes

Servings: 8

Difficulty: Easy

INGREDIENTS

- 2 ½ tbsp Balsamic glaze

- 1 cup Hothouse tomatoes

- 1/3 cup Basil leaves

- ½ cup Mozzarella cheese

- 2 tbsp Olive oil

DIRECTIONS

1. Take tomatoes & mozzarella and make slices of it.

2. Arrange the slices with basil leaves with the alternate pattern on the serving plate.

3. Drizzle it with olive oil.

4. Add balsamic glaze.

5. Sprinkle salt & pepper.

6. Serve and enjoy.

NUTRITION: Calories: 375 cal Fat: 26 g Protein: 20.9 g Carbs: 12.6 g

14. Cabbage and Cucumber Salad

Ready in: 20 minutes

Servings: 3

Difficulty: Easy

INGREDIENTS

- Black pepper

- 3-5 Cucumbers

- 1 cup Mayonnaise

- One cabbage

- Salt

- ½ cup Yogurt

DIRECTIONS

1. Cut cucumbers.

2. Shred cabbage.

3. Transfer both in a large bowl and add yogurt, salt, mayonnaise, and pepper.

4. Mix well to combine all the ingredients.

5. Serve immediately.

6. Enjoy.

NUTRITION: Calories: 143.7 cal Fat: 14.4 g Protein: 1 g Carbs: 3 g

15. Avocado Tuna Salad

Ready in: 15 minutes

Servings: 3

Difficulty: Easy

INGREDIENTS

- 1 tsp salt and pepper

- 15 oz. tuna with oil

- Five sliced avocados

- One sliced cucumber

- One sliced onion

- 2tbsp of lemon juice

- ¼ cup cilantro

- 2 tbsp olive oil

DIRECTIONS

1. Take a large bowl and mix all the ingredients.

2. Drizzle with lemon juice, olive oil, salt, and pepper.

3. Toss well.

4. Serve and enjoy.

NUTRITION: Calories: 304 cal Fat: 20 g Protein: 22 g Carbs: 9 g

Chapter 14: Smoothies Recipes

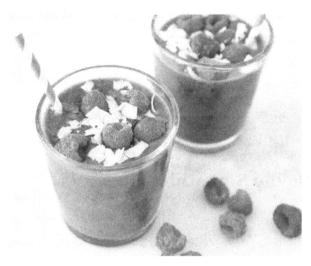

1. Chocolate Coconut Crunch Smoothie

Ready in: 5 minutes

Servings: 2

Difficulty: Easy

INGREDIENTS

- ½ tbsp butter

- 4 oz coconut milk

- 8 oz almond milk

- Salt to taste

- 2 tbsp coconut oil

- 2 tbsp cocoa powder

DIRECTIONS

1. Add all the ingredients to a food processor and blend to get a smooth, creamy mixture.

2. Serve and enjoy it.

NUTRITION: Calories: 222 cal Fat: 23.1 g Protein: 2.5 g Carbs: 5.4 g

2. Rose and Pistachio Smoothie

Ready in: 5 minutes

Servings: 2

Difficulty: Easy

INGREDIENTS

- ¼ rose essence

- 1 L milk

- ½ cup sugar

- 1 cup ice cream

- ¼ cup pistachios

DIRECTIONS

1. Add all the ingredients in a food processor except for ice cream and blend to get a smooth, creamy mixture.

2. Serve with an ice cream scoop and enjoy it.

NUTRITION: Calories: 679 kcal Fat: 47.9 g Protein: 26.8 g Carbs: 45.3 g

3. Banana Pecan Smoothie

Ready in: 5 minutes

Servings: 2

Difficulty: Easy

INGREDIENTS

- ½ tsp cinnamon

- 1 ½ cups vanilla yogurt

- 1 cup ice

- Two sliced bananas

- ½ cup chopped pecans, toasted

- 1 tbsp honey

- ½ cup milk

DIRECTIONS

1. Add all the ingredients to a food processor and blend to get a smooth, creamy mixture.

2. Serve and enjoy it.

NUTRITION: Calories: 390 cal Fat: 24 g Protein: 11 g Carbs: 39 g

4. Turmeric Milkshake

Ready in: 8 minutes

Servings: 2

Difficulty: Easy

INGREDIENTS

- ¼ cinnamon

- 1 cup coconut milk

- 1 ½ banana

- ½ cup almond milk

- Black pepper to taste

- 2 tsp turmeric

- ¼ cup grated coconut

- 1 tbsp almond butter

- ¼ tsp vanilla extract

- 2 tbsp chia seeds

- Salt to taste

DIRECTIONS

1. Add all the ingredients to a food processor and blend to get a smooth, creamy mixture.

2. Serve and enjoy it.

NUTRITION: Calories: 351 cal Fat: 35.2 g Protein: 1.7 g Carbs: 5.5 g

5. Hot Apple Cider Vinegar Tea

Ready in: 5 minutes

Servings: 1

Difficulty: Easy

INGREDIENTS

- 2 tsp liquid stevia

- 1 ½ tbsp apple cider vinegar

- 1 tsp cinnamon

- 1 tbsp lemon juice

- 2 cup boiling water

DIRECTIONS

1. Add all the ingredients to a food processor and blend to get a smooth, creamy mixture.

2. Serve and enjoy it before going to bed.

NUTRITION: Calories: 100 cal Fat: 0 g Protein: 0.3 g Carbs: 22 g

6. Chocolate Milkshake

Ready in: 5 minutes

Servings: 1

Difficulty: Easy

INGREDIENTS

- 1 tsp diced roasted hazelnuts

- Five marshmallows

- 1 tbsp chocolate spread

- 1 cup ice cream, chocolate

- 2 cups milk

- ½ cup whipped cream

DIRECTIONS

1. Cover the glass from inside with the chocolate spread.

2. Add chocolate spread, ice cream, and milk in blender and blend.

3. Transfer the mixture into serving glasses.

4. Garnish with marshmallows, whipped cream, and hazelnuts.

5. Serve and enjoy it.

NUTRITION: Calories: 671 cal Fat: 37 g Protein: 15 g Carbs: 70 g

7. Hurricane Cocktail

Ready in: 5 minutes

Servings: 2

Difficulty: Easy

INGREDIENTS

- 2 tsp grenadine

- 1 cup rum, white and dark

- 1/3 cup orange juice

- One passion fruit

- 1 ½ tbsp lemon juice

- Cocktail cherries for garnishing

- 1/3 cup sugar syrup

- Orange slices for garnishing

DIRECTIONS

1. Add all the ingredients to a food processor and blend to get a smooth, creamy mixture.

2. Serve and enjoy it.

NUTRITION: Calories: 215 kcal Fat: 0 g Protein: 0.5 g Carbs: 24 g

8. Mai Tai Cocktail

Ready in: 5 minutes

Servings: 1

Difficulty: Easy

INGREDIENTS

- ½ oz orgeat

- 1 ½ oz pineapple juice

- ¾ oz orange curacao

- 2 oz rum, dark and light

- ¾ oz lime juice

DIRECTIONS

1. Add all the ingredients to a food processor and blend to get a smooth, creamy mixture.

2. Serve and enjoy it.

NUTRITION: Calories: 262 kcal Fat: 1 g Protein: 1 g Carbs: 24 g

9. Pistachio Smoothie

Ready in: 10 minutes

Servings: 2

Difficulty: Easy

INGREDIENTS

- One banana

- 2 cups crushed ice

- 1/3 cup pistachios

- 2 tsp sugar

- 1 cup milk

- 8 oz vanilla yogurt

DIRECTIONS

1. Add all the ingredients to a food processor and blend to get a smooth mixture.

2. Serve and enjoy it.

NUTRITION: Calories: 801 cal Fat: 61 g Protein: 27 g Carbs: 49 g

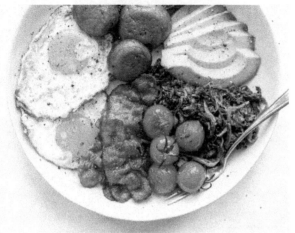

1. Cheesy Bread Bake

Ready in: 20 mins

Servings: 5

Difficulty: Easy

INGREDIENTS

- One loaf of any bread

- 1 cup mozzarella cheese (shredded)

- ¼ cup butter

- 2 cups cheddar cheese (shredded)

- ¼ cup of mayonnaise

- Two cloves minced garlic

- ¼ cup green onion, finely chopped

DIRECTIONS

1. Mix garlic and butter in a bowl.

2. Mix green onion and cheese separately in a bowl, and then add mayonnaise to it.

3. Add this mixture of cheese into butter and garlic mixture.

4. Spread the mixture on the bread loaf.

5. Preheat the broiler and place bread for 4 to 5 mins.

6. Let it cool for 5 mins and then slice it with a knife

7. Serve it.

NUTRITION: Calories: 199 cal Fat: 14 g Protein: 6 g Carbs: 25 g

2. Cocoa Oatmeal

Ready in: 8 minutes

Servings: 1

Difficulty: Easy

INGREDIENTS

- ½ tsp vanilla extract

- ¾ cup oats

- Sea salt to taste

- 1 1/3 cup almond milk

- 2 tsp brown sugar

- ½ sliced banana

- 2tpsp cocoa powder

DIRECTIONS

1. Combine all the ingredients in a mixing bowl.

2. Cook it for 5 to 8 minutes at the medium flame with frequent stirring.

3. Pour it in a bowl and enjoy it.

NUTRITION: Calories: 360 cal Fat: 9 g Protein: 12 g Carbs: 67 g

3. Cheddar Hash Browns

Ready in: 50 minutes

Servings: 11

Difficulty: Medium

INGREDIENTS

- 1 cup parmesan cheese, grated

- 30 oz. hash brown, shredded and frozen potatoes

- 2 cups cheddar cheese, shredded

- Two cans of condensed cream (potato soup)

- 2 cups of sour cream

DIRECTIONS

1. Take half of the cheddar cheese and all the remaining ingredients in a mixing bowl.

2. Pour this mixture into a baking dish.

3. Now add the left amount of cheddar cheese.

4. Heat oven to 340° and bake it for 43 mins.

5. Leave it for 10 mins before serving.

NUTRITION: Calories: 305 cal Fat: 17 g Protein: 11 g Carbs: 22 g

4. Banana and Blueberry Oats

Prep in: 10 minutes

Chill in: 8 hour

Servings: 1

Difficulty: difficult

INGREDIENTS

- 1 tsp vanilla

- ½ cup oats

- 1/3 cup sliced banana

- ½ cup milk

- ½ cup blueberries

DIRECTIONS

1. Mix vanilla, milk, and oats in a bowl.

2. Add blueberries and banana layers over it.

3. Refrigerate it for 8 hours.

4. Serve and enjoy.

NUTRITION: Calories: 320 cal Fat: 5 g Protein: 13 g Carbs: 65 g

5. Trout Frittata

Ready in: 25 minutes

Servings: 5

Difficulty: Easy

INGREDIENTS

- ½ tsp salt

- ¼ cup basil leaves

- Eight eggs

- 4 oz. trout

- ½ cup cream, heavy

- Ten sliced tomatoes

- 3tpsp olive oil

- One chopped shallot

- One chopped bulb fennel

- 2 oz. cheese

DIRECTIONS

6. In a bowl, whisk cream and egg till the mixture becomes smooth.

7. Take a skillet and heat it, then adds oil and heat for 1 minute.

8. Add shallots, fennel, and salt and cook for 4 min.

9. Add trout and tomatoes and cook for 1 min.

10. Bring the cooked egg up by scraping the pan bottom with a spatula.

11. Repeat it twice.

12. Sprinkle basil and cheese on top.

13. Broil the frittata in the preheated broiler for 4 to 5 min.

14. Cool and serve it.

NUTRITION: Calories: 190 cal Fat: 13 g Protein: 15 g Carbs: 1.5 g

6. Sausage and Peppers

Ready in: 60 minutes

Servings: 6

Difficulty: Medium

INGREDIENTS

- ¼ cup diced basil

- 3tbsp olive oil

- Salt as required

- Three bell peppers

- 1tbsp vinegar

- Pepper to taste

- Two minced garlic cloves

- Six sliced sausages

- 2tbsp oregano, dried

- One sliced onion

- 1tbsp red pepper, crushed

DIRECTIONS

15. Whisk red pepper, oil, oregano, vinegar, and garlic in a bowl.

16. Add onions and peppers in a bowl and top with sausages.

17. Bake it in preheated oven for 45 mins at 400°.

18. Top it with basil and enjoy.

NUTRITION: Calories: 208.3 cal Fat: 9.2 g Protein: 17.7 g Carbs: 12.5 g

7. Cheese and Sausage Breakfast

Ready in: 15 minutes

Servings: 4

Difficulty: Easy

INGREDIENTS

- Six eggs

- ¾ cup cheese, shredded

- ¾ cup milk

- Six pork sausage

DIRECTIONS

1. Deep fry sausages in the pan over medium flame.

2. Slice them into small pieces.

3. Whisk milk and eggs in a bowl.

4. Take a skillet and pour eggs in it, then add cheese and cook.

5. When eggs are cooked, stir them in sausage.

6. Serve and enjoy.

NUTRITION: Calories: 313 cal Fat: 23.2 g Protein: 22.5 g Carbs: 3 g

8. Creamy Zucchini

Ready in: 20 minutes

Servings: 6

Difficulty: Easy

INGREDIENTS

- Cheese, shredded

- 1 ½ tsp garlic, minced

- Four chopped zucchini

- 6 oz. cubed cream cheese

- 1/8 tsp pepper, ground

- 2tbsp olive oil

- ¼ tsp salt

- Nutmeg, ground

- 1 cup cream

DIRECTIONS

1. Sauté zucchini in a pan for 4-5 mins.

2. Add garlic in it and cook for a minute.

3. Now drain zucchini from the pan.

4. In the same pan, add cream and cream cheese cook over low flame.

5. Add zucchini mixture into this pan and cook with stirring.

6. Sprinkle it with nutmeg, pepper, and salt.

7. Serve and enjoy.

NUTRITION: Calories: 211.6 cal Fat: 18.9 g Protein: 4.4 g Carbs: 7.6 g

9. Kale and Cheese

Ready in: 15 minutes

Servings: 8

Difficulty: Easy

INGREDIENTS

- 2 cups Cheddar cheese, shredded

- Two bunch of kale

DIRECTIONS

1. Wash and dry kale and dice it into thin slices.

2. Spray cooking oil on baking sheets.

3. Spread kale over baking sheets and top it with cheddar cheese.

4. Bake it in the preheated oven at 425 F for 10-12 mins.

5. Serve and enjoy.

NUTRITION: Calories: 170 cal Fat: 10.1 g Protein: 10.7 g Carbs: 11.6 g

10. Tomato Quiche

Ready in: 1 hour 10 minutes

Servings: 8

Difficulty: Difficult

INGREDIENTS

- 1 ½ cup cream

- Dough

- Four eggs

- 1 cup onion, chopped

- 2 cups cheese

- 1 tsp salt

- 2tbsp butter

- ¼ tsp thyme, dried

- Four chopped tomatoes

- ¼ tsp pepper

DIRECTIONS

1. Roll the dough and transfer it to the baking dish as a crust.

2. Sauté onions in a pan over medium flame and thyme, salt, tomatoes, and pepper in it.

3. Cook it for 10-12 mins over medium flame.

4. In a baking dish, add cheese and top it with tomatoes and sprinkle the remaining cheese.

5. Beat eggs in a separate bowl and pour it.

6. Bake it in the preheated oven at 425 Fahrenheit for 10-12 mins.

7. Reduce the heat of the oven to 325 Fahrenheit and bake it for 40 mins.

NUTRITION: Calories: 484 cal Fat: 35 g Protein: 15 g Carbs: 7 g

11. Salmon Quiche

Ready in: 1 hour 10 minutes

Servings: 8

Difficulty: difficult

INGREDIENTS

- 1tbsp butter

- ¼ tsp salt

- One pastry shell, unbaked

- 2 cups cream

- One chopped onion

- Five eggs

- 2 cups cheese, shredded

- Parsley

- One can salmon

DIRECTIONS

1. In a pan, add butter and sauté onions in it.

2. Add cheese to the crust and then top t with onion and salmon.

3. Whisk salt, cream, and onion in a bowl and pour it over the salmon mixture.

4. Now, bake it for 50 mins at 350 Fahrenheit.

5. Serve and enjoy.

NUTRITION (per slice): Calories: 448 cal Fat: 29 g Protein: 26 g
Carbs: 18 g

Chapter 16: Lunch Recipes

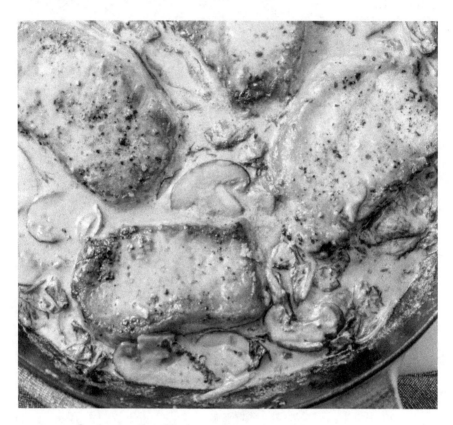

1. Lamb Meatballs

Ready in: 50 minutes

Servings: 4

Difficulty: medium

INGREDIENTS

- One egg, chopper

- 1 lb lamb

- 2 tbsp crushed parsley

- Three bulbs chopped garlic.

- 1 tsp cumin

- 2 tsp crushed oregano

- ½ tsp black pepper

- 1 tsp salt

- 3 tbsp olive oil

- ¼ tsp red chili powder

Green Goddess sauce

- 1 ½ cup basil

- 1 ½ cup Yogurt

- ½ cup mayonnaise

- ¼ crushed chives

- ½ parsley

- 1 tbsp lemon juice

- ¼ cup oregano

- Black pepper to taste

- Two bulb garlic

- Salt to taste

DIRECTIONS

1. Preheat the oven to 425 Fahrenheit. Using parchment paper, cover a large baking sheet. Combine all the ingredients except for sauce in a bowl.

2. Make meatballs out of the batter.

3. Drizzle oil and bake for 20 mins.

4. In the meantime, whisk the ingredients of the sauce in a bowl and blend.

5. Serve the meatballs warm with a dipping sauce made from the green goddess.

NUTRITION: Calories: 670 kcal Fat: 198 g Protein: 48 g Carbs: 67 g

2. Lamb Chops with Garlic Mint Sauce

Ready in: 21 minutes

Servings: 4

Difficulty: Easy

INGREDIENTS

- ½ tsp salt

- 3 lb slice Lamb

- ½ tsp black pepper

- 2 tbsp olive oil

- Mint and Garlic sauce

- 1 tbsp vinegar

- Three bulbs garlic

- 1 tbsp sesame oil

- 2 tbsp soy sauce

- 2 tbsp crushed mint

- ½ tsp red pepper

DIRECTIONS

1. Ready the barbecue and the lamb: Preheat the grill pan over high heat until nearly smoking. All sides of the lamb chops should be seasoned with salt and pepper.

2. Make the sauce: In a mixing cup, whisk together all of the sauce ingredients.

3. Barbecue: Coat or clean the grill pan with cooking spray or olive oil. Sear the chops for 2 mins in a hot grill pan, then flip them and heat for 3 1/2 mins on med or 2 1/2 mins on med-rare.

4. To eat, drizzle a generous amount of garlic and mint sauce over each chop.

3. Potato and Beet Hash with Poached Eggs and Greens

Ready in: 45 minutes

Servings: 5

Difficulty: Easy

INGREDIENTS

- 2 cups chopped gold potato

- 2 tbsp olive oil

- 1 cup crushed onion

- 1 tbsp crushed sage

- 2 cups chopped sweet potato

- One cup cooked red beets.

- Three bulbs chopped garlic

- ½ tsp black pepper

- ½ tsp salt

- Four eggs

- 5 tsp wine vinegar

- 6 cups radicchio

- ½ tsp mustard

DIRECTIONS

1. Heat on med heat 1 tbsp oil in a large nonstick skillet. Add the onion to the skillet and roast for 5 mins, or till golden brown and tender. Cook, stirring regularly, for 25 mins or until potatoes are soft, adding two tsp sage and garlic as desired. Cook for 10 mins, stirring regularly, after adding the beets, 1/4 tsp salt, and 1/4 tsp pepper.

2. Fill a large skillet two-thirds full of water. Reduce to low heat after bringing to boil and proceed to cook. One tbsp of vinegar Each egg should be split into a custard cup and carefully poured into the pan. Cook for 3 mins, or until cooked to your taste. Using a slotted spoon, scrape the eggs from the pan. Evenly scatter 1/2 tsp sage over eggs.

3. Inside a large mixing bowl, beat together the remaining 1 tbsp oil, 2 tsp vinegar, 1/4 tsp salt, 1/2 tsp sage, 1/4 tsp pepper, and mustard. Toss in the frisée to coat. Serve with eggs and hash.

NUTRITION: Calories: 329 kcal Fat: 11.5 g Protein: 11.7 g Carbs: 45.5 g

4. Moroccan Lamb

Ready in: 45 minutes

Servings: 4

Difficulty: Medium

INGREDIENTS

- 3 tsp cinnamon

- 500g lamb

- 2 tsp paprika

- Olive oil

- Two tomatoes, sliced

- 1 tbsp crushed parsley

- ½ tsp chopped garlic

DIRECTIONS

1. Inside a large frying pan, heat the oil. Cook the lamb completely on both sides without using any additional oil. Add the spices and simmer for another min or until fragrant.

2. Bring the tomatoes and parsley to a boil, then reduce to low heat and roast for 30 mins, or till your lamb is tender. Serve with more parsley on top.

NUTRITION: Calories:350 kcal Fat: 22 g Protein: 27 g Carbs: 13 g

5. Paleo Lamb Meatloaf

Ready in: 110 minutes

Servings: 6

Difficulty: Difficult

INGREDIENTS

- ½ chopped onion

- 2 tbsp olive oil

- Salt to taste

- Two chopped celery ribs

- One ¼ lb lamb

- ½ tsp chili

- ½ cup coconut flour

- Two chopped eggs

- ½ tsp parsley

- 1/3 cup tomato ketchup

- ½ tsp rosemary

- ½ tsp basil

- 1 tsp cumin

- ½ tsp thyme

- ½ cup goat feta

- 2 tsp coconut sauce

DIRECTIONS

1. Preheat the oven to 400 Fahrenheit. Using parchment paper, baking pan such that it stretches over the sides and forms handles.

2. In a med sautés pan, heat the olive oil over med-low heat. Cook, occasionally stirring, until the onions and celery are soft for about 10-15 mins.

3. Combine all the remaining ingredients and stir well. Mix thoroughly. Fill baking tray halfway with the batter. Ketchup can be spread on top.

4. Place the baking pan inside and Preheat the oven. To prevent the top from cracking, place a pan of hot water on the oven rack below the meatloaf pan. Preheat the oven and bake for one hour.

5. Serve and enjoy it.

NUTRITION: Calories: 215 kcal Fat: 14 g Protein: 17 g Carbs: 5 g

6. Beef & Walnut Stir Fry with Veggie Rice

Ready in: 20 minutes

Servings: 2

Difficulty: Easy

INGREDIENTS

*   One red chili powder

- 1 tbsp coconut oil

- 2 tsp honey

- Two steaks, slice

- 3 tbsp walnuts, toast

- Three sliced onion

- 2 tsp coconut oil

- ½ cup basil

- Six broccoli cut into pieces

- Four cauliflower cut into pieces.

- Black pepper to taste.

- ½ lemon juice

- Salt to taste

DIRECTIONS

1. In a wok, until hot, heat half of the oil.

2. Cook for 2-3 mins with the pepper before withdrawing from the wok.

3. Fried for 3 mins the beef in the remaining oil, then the peppers, spring onions, & walnuts, along with soy or tamari sauce & honey is added.

4. Cook for 1 min, stirring well.

5. Season to taste with pepper and salt before mixing in the basil leaves just before eating.

6. Blitz the cauliflower and broccoli until they are finely chopped.

7. Heat the coconut oil in a large skillet, and cook the vegetables for 5 mins, stirring continuously.

8. Only before serving the beef, season it and add the lemon zest and juice.

NUTRITION: Calories: 731 kcal Fat: 25 g Protein: 51 g Carbs: 17 g

7. Loaded Lebanese Rice: Yahweh

Ready in: 50 minutes

Servings: 5

Difficulty: Easy

INGREDIENTS

- Olive oil

- 1 ½ cups Grain rice

- 1 lb. beef

- One sliced onion

- ½ tsp garlic paste.

- One ¾ tsp allspice

- Pepper to taste

- ¾ tsp cinnamon

- ¾ ground cloves

- Salt to taste

- ½ cup pine

- ½ cup sliced parsley

- ½ cup raisins

- ½ cup almonds

DIRECTIONS

1. Soak the rice in chilly water for 15 mins.

2. In a pot, heat oil. Add cleaved red onions, cook on med-high warmth momentarily; at that point, the ground beef is added. Season the mixture of meat with allspice (one ¼ tsp), minced garlic, ground cloves (½ tsp), ground cinnamon (½ tsp), salt, & pepper. Cook until the meat is completely caramelized (8-10 mins).

3. Top the meat with rice. The rice is seasoned with salt and the rest of the allspice, cinnamon, and ground cloves. Add one tbsp of olive oil to cover the rice and 2 ½ cups of water.

4. Turn warmth to high and carry the fluid to a moving bubble. Let bubble until the fluid has fundamentally diminished (see picture beneath).

5. Now go warmth to low and cover; let cook for 20 mins or until dampness has been ingested and the rice is not. Remove from warmth and put in a safe spot for 10 mins.

6. Uncover the rice pot and spot an enormous round serving platter on the launch of the rice pot. Cautiously the pot substance is flipped on the platter.

7. Garnish with almonds, toasted pine nuts, raisins, and parsley.

NUTRITION: Calories: 389 kcal Fat: 30.9 g Protein: 20.1 g Carbs: 11.1 g

8. Corned Beef & Cauli Hash

Ready in: 30 minutes

Servings: 4

Difficulty: Easy

INGREDIENTS

- 3 cups of cooked corned beef

- One head of chopped fresh cauliflower

- 1/2 yellow onion, chopped

- 1 tbsp olive oil

- salt and pepper

- 1 tsp Cajun seasoning

- Optional: 4 eggs

- Garnish: Fresh chopped parsley

DIRECTIONS

1. Take a medium-sized skillet and heat olive oil in it.

2. Take water in a bowl and put some chopped cauliflower.

3. Put the bowl in the microwave for 3-5 minutes.

4. Take a skillet and brown the onion in it over medium flame.

5. Add 2-3 tbsp of water.

6. Once cauliflower is steamed, let it set for some time.

7. Mix the cauliflower and seasonings in skillet and mix.

8. Now add the beef and cook for 3-5 minutes.

9. Put some salt and pepper according to taste and garnish with parsley and top with eggs.

10. Serve and enjoy.

NUTRITION: Calories: 221 Cal Fat: 14 g Protein: 23 g Carbs: 2 g

9. Baked Sea Bass with Pesto, Zucchini, and Carrots

Ready in: 25-35 minutes

Servings: 4

Difficulty: Easy

INGREDIENTS

- 3/4 tsp salt

- Four sea-bass fillets, about 1 inch thick

- 1/2 tsp fresh-ground black pepper

- 1/4 cup of pesto, store-bought/homemade

- Three carrots, grated

- One zucchini, grated

- 2 tbsps olive oil

- 1/4 cup of dry white wine

DIRECTIONS

1. Take a baking dish, place Al-foil over it, and heat the microwave to 400.

2. Rub fish with pepper and salt.

3. Spread it with pesto. Cover it with carrots and top with zucchini. Gather around the foil and drizzle with olive oil. Make a sealed package and put it on the baking sheet.

4. Bake it for 10-15 minutes. Open the package and transfer them to the plates.

5. Enjoy.

NUTRITION: Calories: 265 Cal Fat: 10 g Protein: 34 g Carbs: 9 g

10. Sriracha Tuna Chili

Ready in: 20 minutes

Servings: 5

Difficulty: Easy

INGREDIENTS

- 2 Tbsps Canola Oil

- 2 cups of Tuna

- 15 oz fried Vegetables

- 16 oz Kidney Beans

- 1.25 oz Chili Seasoning

- 15 oz Beans

- 10 Tbsps Salsa

- 10 Tsp Chili Sauce

- 50g Sriracha

- 28 oz Crushed Tomatoes

- 2 Tsp Garlic

DIRECTIONS

1. Take beans in a bowl and rinse well.

2. Drain the tuna.

3. Take a pan and heat olive oil on a medium flame.

4. Once the pan is heated, add the remaining ingredients to it and mix well.

5. Cook for 15-20 minutes and keep moving with a spatula after regular intervals.

6. Serve and enjoy.

NUTRITION: Calories: 380 Cal Fat: 6 g Protein: 32 g Carbs: 49.5 g

11. Poached Cod with Tomato and Saffron

Ready in: 10-15 minutes

Servings: 4

Difficulty: Easy

INGREDIENTS

- 2 tbsps olive oil

- Two mashed garlic cloves

- 1 tsp crushed pepper

- 14.5-oz tomatoes

- 1/4 cup of wine

- Two bay leaves

- Saffron threads Pinch

- Kosher salt, freshly ground pepper

- 4 oz skinless cod fillets

DIRECTIONS

1. Take a skillet and heat olive oil over medium flame.

2. Add garlic & Aleppo pepper to it. Cook for 3-5 minutes.

3. Crush the tomatoes with hands and add with bay leaves and a 1-4th cup of water. Cook it and bring a boil.

4. Season with salt and pepper.

5. Transfer cod to bowls and spoon with the poaching liquid.

7. Enjoy.

NUTRITION: Calories: 429 Cal Fat: 15 g Protein: 37 g Carbs: 38 g

12. Garlic Parmesan Roasted Radishes

Ready in: 50 minutes

Servings: 4

Difficulty: Easy

INGREDIENTS

- 2 tsp chopped rosemary

- Two bundle radishes

- Four bulbs chopped garlic

- Two olive oil

- 2 tbsp butter

- ¼ cup cheese

- Salt to taste

DIRECTIONS

1. Up to 400 Fahrenheit, preheat the oven and cover a baking sheet with parchment paper.

2. Combine radishes, melted butter, minced garlic, rosemary, cinnamon, and pepper in a mixing bowl. Toss all together thoroughly. 45 mins of roasting

3. Coat all of the radishes with parmesan cheese. Cook for another 5 mins, or until golden and crisp.

4. When finished, serve the roasted radishes as a side dish or as a full meal.

NUTRITION: Calories: 87 kcal Fat: 7 g Protein: 2 g Carbs: 2 g

13. Balsamic Roasted Cabbage Steaks

Ready in: 40minutes

Servings: 6

Difficulty: Medium

INGREDIENTS

- ½ tsp mustard

- ¼ cup olive oil

- 2 tbsp vinegar

- ½ tsp honey

- One bulb chopped garlic

- Parsley as required

- Salt to taste

- Black pepper to taste

DIRECTIONS

1. Preheat the oven to 400 Fahrenheit.

2. Gently oil a baking sheet and set it aside.

3. Cut the cabbage's bottom (root) and set it up on the cutting board with the flat end facing up; slice into 1-inch thick slices.

4. Place cabbage slices on a baking sheet that has already been prepared.

5. In a mixing cup, add the extra virgin olive oil, balsamic vinegar, mustard, garlic, sugar, salt, and pepper.

6. Spray all sides of the cabbage steaks with the prepared balsamic glaze.

7. Roast for 20 to 25 mins, or until the potatoes are crispy and tender.

NUTRITION: Calories: 87 kcal Fat: 9 g Protein: 0.5 g Carbs: 1 g

14. Grilled eggplant, tomato, and Mint Salad

Ready in: 40 minutes

Servings: 4

Difficulty: Medium

INGREDIENTS

- Salt to taste

- Two eggplants cut into a piece.

- Olive oil as required

- Black pepper to taste

- 2 tbsp lemon juice

- One bulb chopped garlic

- 1 tbsp sugar

- 1 tbsp red chili

- ¼ cup crushed mint

- 6 tbsp olive oil

- ½ grape tomatoes

- ½ cup crushed parsley

DIRECTIONS

1. Salt the eggplant generously and spread it out on a towel-lined baking sheet in a single layer. After 30 mins, blot the eggplant dry and spray generously with olive oil on both sides; set aside.

2. In a chimney starter, light 6 quarts of charcoal and heat until the coals are filled with a fine grey ash coating, about 15 mins. Cover half of the barbecue with charcoal, cover with the grill grate, and heat for 5 mins. Clean the grate with a scraper.

3. Grill eggplant for 2-4 mins, or until browned. Cook for another 3 mins until the eggplant is finely browned and tender.

4. To make the emulsion, mix the garlic, cayenne, lemon juice, pepper, sugar, a pinch of salt, and 6 tbsps olive oil.

5. Cut eggplant to make it half-inch-wide strips, and with dressing, toss it.

NUTRITION: Calories: 310 kcal Fat: 27.6 g Protein: 2.9 g Carbs:16.3 g

Chapter 17: Dinner Recipes

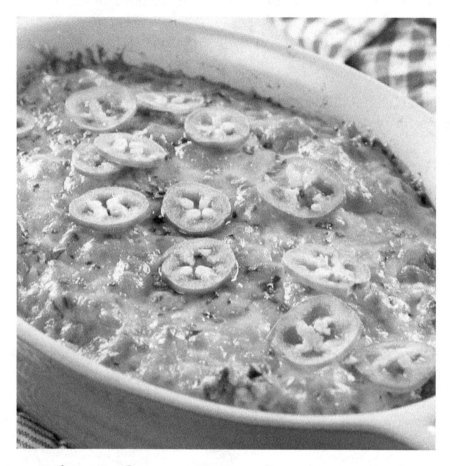

1. Cajun Crabmeat Casserole

Ready in: 65 minutes

Servings: 6

Difficulty: Medium

INGREDIENTS

- 2 ½ tbsp butter

- 1/3 cup crushed celery

- 1/3 cups sliced scallion

- ½ cup green chili paste

- 6 tbsp mayonnaise

- Two cloves garlic paste

- 1 tbsp mustard

- 2 tsp sauce

- 2 tsp crushed parsley

- Salt to taste

- 1 tsp tabasco sauce

- 1 tsp cayenne pepper

- One egg

- 1 cup cream

- 1 lb lump crabmeat

- Paprika to taste

DIRECTIONS

1. Add butter to a saucepan and melt it at medium heat. Add celery, garlic, scallions, and bell pepper in it and cook it for a time until vegetables are tender.

2. Take the pan from heat and add other ingredients like mustard, mayonnaise, parsley, Worcestershire sauce, salt, cayenne, and Tabasco and stir them until completely blended.

3. Add this mixture to the egg and mix them smoothly.

4. Now add crabmeat and pour this mixture into the casserole dish.

5. Drizzle cream throughout the mixture

6. Place this mixture in the oven that is already heated at 350°F and bake it for 20 minutes.

7. Serve immediately.

NUTRITION: Calories: 450 kcal Fat: 51 g Protein: 20 g Carbs: 31 g

2. Tuna Cauliflower Rice

Ready in: 15 minutes

Servings: 5

Difficulty: Easy

INGREDIENTS

- 1 tbsp coconut oil

- 2 tsp chopped Ginger

- One cloves crushed garlic

- 1 /4 cauliflower cut into slice

- Two crushed onion

- 1 cup chopped capsicum

- One crushed chili

- 2 tbsp coconut

- 2 tbsp crushed coriander

- 3 lb tuna

- 1 tbsp soy sauce

- 1 tbsp lemon juice

DIRECTIONS

1. Make a cauliflower recipe, make its small florets and then process it in a food processor, converting it into fine rice.

2. Take a frying pan, add olive oil to it, and heat it. Then add other ingredients like cauliflower, capsicum, garlic, ginger, chili, spring onions.

3. Now cook it for 1-2 minutes.

4. Now add tuna, coconut, and fresh lemon juice and cook it.

5. To make it tasty, season it with tamari. Serve it while hot.

NUTRITION: Calories: 108 kcal Fat: 3 g Protein: 7 g Carbs: 9 g

3. Crawfish Boil Recipe

Ready in: 60 minutes

Servings: 5

Difficulty: Medium

INGREDIENTS

- 3 lb crawfish

- 6 oz crawfish shrimp

- 10 cups water

- 2 tbsp Cajun seasoning

- One clove garlic

- 14 oz sausage

- 1 tbsp Lemon Pepper seasoning

- One minced lemon

- Three ears corn

- 13 oz chopped red potatoes

DIRECTIONS

1. Boil water in a pot.

2. Mix in seasoning, crab, lemon pepper, and shrimp and let it cook.

3. Stir in the potatoes, garlic, sausage, corn, and lemon slices. Cover and let it cook for 10 minutes.

4. Transfer the crawfish into the pot and cook for 3-4 minutes, with the lid covered.

5. Turn off the heat and let the crawfish soak for 10 minutes.

6. Remove all the ingredients using a strainer and serve immediately. Discard the crawfish boil water.

NUTRITION: Calories: 317 kcal Fat: 18 g Protein: 16 g Carbs: 22 g

4. Thai Coconut Clams

Ready in: 30 minutes

Servings: 5

Difficulty: Easy

INGREDIENTS

- One lemon cut into slices

- 1 tbsp coconut oil

- One stalk lemongrass

- Three chopped shallots

- ½ cup vegetable soup

- Two jalapeno peppers

- 1 tbsp chopped ginger

- 2 tbsp sauce

- ½ cup coconut milk

- 1 tbsp sugar

- 2 lb scrubbed

- One crushed scallion

- Salt to taste

- ½ cup crushed cilantro leaves

DIRECTIONS

1. For this recipe, take a pressure cooker, add oil to it and boil it. Then add sauté and shallots and cook for 3-5 minutes until they become soft and brown at the edges.

2. While cooking, take a lemongrass stalk and remove its outer layers and bruise its core.

3. Take the instant pot and add ginger, jalapeños, fish sauce, brown sugar, and lemongrass stalk. Continuously stir it and make sure that brown sugar is completely dissolved. Then add coconut milk and stir it again for 5 minutes and simmer.

4. Finally, add clams and cook it at low heat for 1-2 minutes. If any claim is not open, remove it. Taste it and add pepper and salt to make it tastier.

5. Serve clams in bowls.

NUTRITION: Calories: 233 kcal Fat: 10 g Protein: 12.5 g Carbs: 18 g

5. Lobster Chili

Ready in: 35 minutes

Servings: 5

Difficulty: Medium

INGREDIENTS

- 2 ½ lb meat

- Six chopped bacon

- Four cloves chopped garlic

- Two chopped onion

- Two crushed jalapeno pepper

- 3 tbsp red chili

- 2 cups kidney beans

- 6 cup tomatoes paste

- 1 tsp cumin

- Salt to taste

- 1 tsp wine vinegar

- 4 oz green chili

DIRECTIONS

1. Take a pot or an oven and add bacon to it and cook at low to medium heat.

2. Use a slotted spoon to remove bacon from the pot and reserve it while leaving bacon fat in the pot. Do not remove bacon fat.

3. Now add sliced onions in bacon fat and cook it for 3-4 minutes at low heat. or when you notice it has become soft.

4. Now add garlic, chili powder, and jalapeños, stir them and cook for 5-10 minutes.

5. Then add tomatoes, vinegar, beans, cumin oregano, and salt, similarly stir them as well.

6. Cook this mixture for up to 20-30 minutes or when it becomes thicken. Liquid smoke can also be added to give it a smoky flavor.

7. Now it is time to add reserved bacon, Maine Lobster, and green chile. Simmer it for few minutes.

NUTRITION: Calories: 419 kcal Fat: 13.5 g Protein: 7 g Carbs: 50.2 g

6. Lobster Deviled Eggs

Ready in: 68 minutes

Servings: 24

Difficulty: Medium

INGREDIENTS

- 1 tbsp paprika

- 12 eggs, cooked

- 1 ½ tsp mustard

- Crushed chives

- ¾ cup mayonnaise

- ½ tsp black pepper

- Red pepper to taste

- Salt to taste

- 1 cup crushed lobster, cooked

DIRECTIONS

1. To make lobster deviled eggs main ingredients are needed eggs and lobsters. First, using a knife lengthwise, cut the eggs. Take one bowl and a serving plate. Pour egg yolk in the bowl while egg white in the serving plate. Using a fork, mash egg

yolk and add mayonnaise to it. Using a mixer, mix them smoothly. Then add lobster and stir

2. On the top of egg white, spray paprika and chives, cover it, and place it in a freezer. When it is chilled, it is ready to serve.

NUTRITION: Calories: 141 kcal Fat: 11 g Protein: 7 g Carbs: 2 g

7. Steamed Clams in Spicy Tomato Sauce

Ready in: 60 minutes

Servings: 4

Difficulty: Medium

INGREDIENTS

- 1 tsp orange juice

- 4 ½ lb clams

- 1 cup wine

- 2 tbsp olive oil

- One chopped onion

- 28 oz tomatoes juice

- ¼ red chili

- ¼ tsp sugar

- Saffron to taste

- 1 tsp thyme

- Salt to taste

- Olive oil

- 4 tbsp crushed parsley

- Lemon juice

DIRECTIONS

1. Clean the clams with a tiny tool, such as a toothbrush, after rinsing them in many changes of water. Anything that is accessible or has broken shells should be discarded.

1. Spoon the wine into a wide, lidded pan large enough to contain each of the clams. Take to the boil, then minimize to half the original number. Add some clams, cover, and cook for 2-3 mins on high heat, tossing the pan periodically before the clams open. Switch off the sun. Some claims that haven't opened can be discarded.

2. Wash the clams in a strainer onto a container lined with cheesecloth. In different cups, put aside the liquid & the clams. Hold your clams in their shells or cut them, whatever is more practical for serving.

3. In a big, broad, lidded skillet or casserole, heat the olive oil on medium heat & add the shallots. Cook for 3 minutes, stirring regularly, until the vegetables are soft, then incorporate the garlic & red pepper flakes. Cook, stirring continuously for 30 secs to 1 min until it is fragrant, then add the tomatoes with juice, thyme, orange zest, saffron, sugar, and clam liquid. Season with salt & pepper to taste, then bring to a boil over

medium heat for 20-25 mins, stirring regularly, until the mixture has thoroughly cooked & is very fragrant. Season with salt and pepper to taste.

4. Heat the clams in the tomato sauce, stirring continuously. Stir in parsley or cilantro and serve in big soup cups. Drizzle each serving with some olive oil and several drops of lemon juice.

NUTRITION: Calories: 602 kcal Fat: 12 g Protein: 77 g Carbs: 32 g

8. Smoked Cod Pate Platter

Ready in: 15 minutes

Servings: 5

Difficulty: Easy

INGREDIENTS

- 3 tbsp Yoghurt

- Two smoked Cod Fillets

- ½ tbsp lemon juice

To Serve

- Apple coleslaw

- Eight oatcakes

- Four chopped radishes

- Four celery sticks

- Four artichoke

Apple coleslaw

- 100 g chopped cabbage

- 100 ml crème

- One lemon juice

- 1 tsp mustard

- 100 g chopped fennel

- One chopped carrot

DIRECTIONS

1. Take a mixing bowl, add cod in it and mesh it smoothly. Then add yogurt, black pepper, and lemon juice. Using a mixer mesh these ingredients as well as make a chunky paste. Pour this mixture into a serving bowl, and it is ready to serve.

2. This chunky pate can be served along with coleslaw and other ingredients on the serving plate.

3. To prepare coleslaw using a mixer, make a mixture of lemon juice, crème Fraiche, and mustard. Also, add vegetables and fruits like apples.

NUTRITION: Calories: 331 kcal Fat: 12 g Protein: 52 g Carbs: 1 g

9. Herbed Cherry Tomatoes

Ready in: 10 minutes

Servings: 4

Difficulty: Easy

INGREDIENTS

- ½ tsp sugar

- 4 cups cherry tomatoes

- 3 tbsp vinegar

- ¼ cup oil

- ¼ cup minced parsley

- 1 ½ tsp chopped oregano

- 1 ½ tsp chopped basil

- ½ tsp salt

DIRECTIONS

1. Take a bowl, add tomatoes to it, and add salt, pepper and vinegar, basil, oregano, and parsley. Add the tomatoes to it.

2. Serve with lettuce leaves.

NUTRITION: Calories: 56 cal Fat: 5 g Protein: 1 g Carbs: 4 g

10. Garlic Seasoned Vegetable Spinach Russian salad

Ready in: 35 minutes

Servings: 6

Difficulty: Easy

INGREDIENTS

- Two minced garlic clove

- One ¾ cups chicken stock

- 4 cups chopped vegetables

DIRECTIONS

1. Take a pan, add the broth, vegetables, and garlic, cook it until the vegetables get soft and broth get a boil, add the salt and pepper according to taste.

2. Strain the water from the vegetables and serve.

NUTRITION: Calories: 208 cal Fat: 18.3 g Protein: 2.7 g Carbs: 9.8 g

11. Savoy Cabbage with Pine Nuts and Sesame Seeds

Ready in: 25 minutes

Servings: 4

Difficulty: Easy

INGREDIENTS

- 3 tbsp balsamic vinegar

- One savoy cabbage

- One onion

- Salt to taste

- 3 tbsp sesame seeds

- 4 tbsp olive oil

- 3 tbsp pine nuts

- Black pepper to taste

DIRECTIONS

1. Slice the cabbage. Take a pan, boil water with some salt, add the cabbage to it, and blanch.

2. Take onions and dice them into rings, sauté them in the oil with some pinenuts and cook for about 5 minutes. Add the cabbage, pepper, and salt.

3. Drizzle vinegar and garnish it with onions.

4. Serve and enjoy it.

NUTRITION: Calories: 126 kcal Fat: 7 g Protein: 5 g Carbs: 15 g

12. Stuffed Cabbage with Ricotta and Pine Nuts

Ready in: 50 minutes

Servings: 4

Difficulty: Medium

INGREDIENTS

- 1 ½ tbsp sugar

- 2 tbsp butter

- 1/8 cup rice

- 1 ½ oz noodles

- One ¼ cup water

- One cabbage

- Salt to taste

- 1/3 cup roasted pine nuts

- ¼ cup shredded cheese, parmesan

- ¾ cup ricotta

- 1 ½ cup vegetable stock

- 3 tbsp diced basil

- Three minced garlic cloves

- 4 tbsp diced parsley

- Black pepper to taste

DIRECTIONS

1. Take a pan, add butter in it, let it melt, add the pinenut, toss the nuts into the batter, and then add the rice and water. Let it simmer for 10-15 mins.

2. Cut the cabbage and blanch it in saltwater for 5 minutes, and then tap dry.

3. Add 2 tbsp cheese(parmesan), garlic, salt, pepper, basil, and parsley, toss them all. Add this nuts mixture to an ovenproof dish and add cabbage at the top of the nuts and rice mixture. Pour the broth, salt, sugar, and pepper mixture at the top and bake it for 35 minutes until the liquid is evaporated.

NUTRITION: Calories: 963 cal Fat: 48 g Protein: 21 g Carbs: 114 g

13. Red Cabbage with Apple, Pinenuts, and Sultanas

Ready in: 30 minutes

Servings: 5

Difficulty: Easy

INGREDIENTS

- 2 tbsp lime juice

- 3 ½ cups diced cabbage

- One chopped apple

- ½ diced onion

- ¼ cup roasted pine nuts

- Two minced garlic cloves

- ¼ cup sultanas

- Salt to taste

DIRECTIONS

1. Take a large saucepan, add some oil, sauté cabbage, onion, garlic for 5-6 minutes in oil. Sprinkle pepper, salt, verjuice, and water; cook until the water evaporates, and the cabbage is softened.

2. Add the pine nuts sultanas and toss them all and cook for few minutes.

3. Serve and enjoy!

NUTRITION: Calories: 963 kcal Fat: 48 g Protein: 21 g Carbs: 114 g

14. Farfalle with Savoy Cabbage, Pancetta and Mozzarella

Ready in: 35 minutes

Servings: 5

Difficulty: Medium

INGREDIENTS

- 7 oz chopped cheese, mozzarella

- ¼ cup olive oil

- 3 tbsp pine nuts

- ¼ lb diced pancetta

- 2 tsp diced thyme

- One ¾ lb savory cabbage

- One chopped garlic clove

- ¼ cup shredded cheese, parmesan

- Salt to taste

- ½ cup water

- Pepper to taste

- 1 lb farfalle

DIRECTIONS

1. Take one large skillet, add oil and pancetta and fry it till golden. Sieve it and chopped it

2. Toast the pine nuts in a saucepan and put them on a plate now; in the skillet, add thyme and garlic, stir it and put

some cabbage in it, sprinkle pepper, parmesan, salt, and some water, cook it on low heat

3. Boil some farfalle.

4. Add pasta in a pot, put the cabbage, season it with salt, parmesan pepper, pine nuts, pancetta, and leftover olive oil and stir it well till the cheese gets melted.

NUTRITION: Calories: 72 kcal Fat: 11 g Protein: 8 g Carbs: 2 g

15. Lemon, Black Pepper, Pecorino and Cabbage Rice

Ready in: 30 minutes

Servings: 4

Difficulty: Easy

INGREDIENTS

- 2 tbsp lemon juice

- Olive oil as required

- 1 ½ cups rice

- One diced onion

- ½ cup butter

- 1 tsp black pepper

- One ¼ quart boiling water

- ½ grated savoy cabbage

- 3 ½ oz shredded cheese, pecorino

DIRECTIONS

1. Take a large pan, and heat olive oil, sauté onions in the pan till it gets translucent

2. In a pot, add some butter and rice, stir it nicely, add water timely and don't try to turn the high flame stir it until the rice gets completely cooked

3. In rice, add sprinkle pepper, pecorino, lemon zest, and some butter to make it creamy.

4. Serve it warmly

NUTRITION: Calories: 131 kcal Fat: 6 g Protein: 5 g Carbs: 13 g

Chapter 18: Snacks Recipes

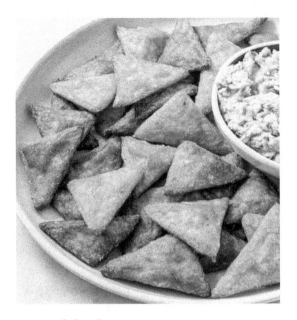

1. Kohl Slaw

Ready in: 75 minutes

Servings: 4

Difficulty: Medium

INGREDIENTS

- Four chopped carrots

- 2 tbsp vinegar

- 1 tbsp nectar

- Black pepper to taste

- 1 tbsp mayonnaise

- 1 tbsp mustard

- Two chopped apple

- Salt to taste

- Two chopped kohlrabi

DIRECTIONS

1. Combine mayonnaise, mustard, vinegar, Dijon, pepper, nectar & salt altogether in the bowl.

2. Mix apples, carrots & kohlrabi into dressing till finely coated. Cove & refrigerate for an hour.

NUTRITION: Calories: 138 kcal Fat: 2.6 g Protein: 3.2 g Carbs: 29.4 g

2. Cornbread Stuffing

Ready in: 60 minutes

Servings: 10

Difficulty: Medium

INGREDIENTS

- Black pepper to taste

- Two stick butter

- 2 tbsp chopped thyme

- 3 tbsp chopped sage

- 2 tbsp chopped parsley

- Salt to taste

- 1 tsp chopped rosemary

Stuffing

- ¾ cup milk

- Two chopped onion

- 9 cups sliced cornbread

- 1 cup chicken soup

- Three chopped celery stalks

- One beaten egg

DIRECTIONS

Cornbread

1. Preheat the oven to 300 Fahrenheit. Mix all the cornbread ingredients all together in a large bowl, then pour into the baking pan.

2. Bake it for 22-24mins / till its top becomes golden brown. Then set it aside to cool (almost overnight). Don't cover.

3. Preheat the oven to 250 Fahrenheit —slice cornbread into 1-inch cubes. You may have almost 7-8 cups cubes, then spread it on a lined baking sheet & bake for 10 min. Set it aside to cool while you'll prepare the stuffing. Set the oven up to 450 Fahrenheit.

Stuffing

1. Whisk broth & eggs in a bowl & set aside.

2. Heat the butter in a large pan on med-high heat. Now add onion, thyme celery, parsley, salt, sage, & pepper & cook for 4 mins till the vegetables begin to get soft. Then squeeze the sausage meat out of casings into the pan. Break it up using a spoon, then add pears & cook till sausage is recently cooked through. Now, pour into broth + egg mixture and any liquid present in the pan. Add toasted cornbread cubes & pecans. Now, gently fold everything all together.

3. Spoon the stuffing into a 9×13baking pan. Bake it for 40mins. Sprinkle it with more parsley (if you want) & serve warm.

NUTRITION: Calories: 354 kcal Fat: 16 g Protein: 14 g Carbs: 40 g

3. Roasted Pumpkin with Nuts and Manchego Cheese

Ready in: 35 minutes

Servings: 5

Difficulty: Easy

INGREDIENTS

- Black pepper to taste

- 2 lb pumpkins

- 2 oz parsley

- Salt to taste

- 3 tbsp olive oil

- ¾ cup hazelnuts

- 2 tsp slice thyme

- 2 tsp crushed Rosemary

- ½ lb cheese

DIRECTIONS

1. Preheat your oven to 400 Fahrenheit.

2. Slice pumpkin into wedges, almost 1" (2,5 cm) thick. You may peel off its skin using a sharp knife / just leave it & peel after it's serving.

3. Brush it with oil on both sides. Pepper & salt to taste. Now place them on the pan & bake it for 15mins / till the wedges of pumpkin get soft.

4. Chop those nuts roughly using a knife & mix with shredded manchego, chopped parsley, & rosemary / dried thyme.

5. Remove pumpkin from oven & spread herbs & nuts on the top & gratinate till cheese starts to melt.

6. Serve along with leafy greens & a splash of olive oil.

NUTRITION: Calories: 722 kcal Fat: 61 g Protein: 26 g Carbs: 18 g

4. Easy Hummus

Ready in: 10 minutes

Servings: 5

Difficulty: Easy

INGREDIENTS

- Paprika paste

- 15 oz chickpeas boiled

- ¼ cup sesame oil

- ¼ cup lemon juice

- 2 tbsp olive oil

- Salt to taste

- ½ tsp cumin

- 3 tbsp water

DIRECTIONS

1. Add all the ingredients in a food processor and blend to get a paste.

2. Transfer the paste in serving bowl.

3. Sprinkle olive oil and paprika and serve.

NUTRITION: Calories: 190 kcal Fat: 11 g Protein: 6 g Carbs: 18 g

5. Roasted Vegetables Tricolored

Ready in: 40 minutes

Servings: 5

Difficulty: Medium

INGREDIENTS

- ½ cup olive oil

- 1 lb Brussels

- 8 oz Mushroom

- 8 oz tomatoes

- Salt to taste

- 1 tsp crushed Rosemary

- ½ tsp black pepper

DIRECTIONS

1. To 200°C, preheat the oven. Rinse & trim all vegetables & peel the outer layer of the Brussels sprouts if needed.

2. Cut the vegetables so they're roughly the same size—place in a 9" baking dish.

3. Add spices & olive oil & mix.

4. Bake for 20 mins or till the vegetables have softened & turned a nice color.

5. Serve as a side dish with meat, chicken, or fish.

NUTRITION: Calories: 208 kcal Fat: 18 g Protein: 4 g Carbs: 6 g

6. Thai Curry Cabbage

Ready in: 30 minutes

Servings: 5

Difficulty: Easy

INGREDIENTS

- 1 tbsp sesame seeds oil

- 3 tbsp coconut oil

- 2 lb crushed cabbage

- 1 tbsp Thai red Curry

- Salt to taste

DIRECTIONS

1. Heat coconut oil in a wok over a high flame. Add curry paste & stir for a min. Add cabbage.

2. Sauté till the cabbage begins to turn golden brown, but still is a little chewy. Stir thoroughly & lower the heat towards the end.

3. Salt to taste. Add sesame oil & sauté for another 1–2 mins & serve.

NUTRITION: Calories: 181 kcal Fat: 13 g Protein: 3 g Carbs: 8 g

7. Pizza Fat Bombs

Ready in: 2 hours 45 minutes

Servings: 6

Difficulty: Difficult

INGREDIENTS

- 4 ounces of cream cheese softened

- ¼ cup of chopped pepperoni

- ¼ cup of chopped black olives

- 2 Tbsps chopped fresh basil

- 2 Tbsps shredded Parmesan cheese

- 2 Tbsps pizza sauce no-sugar-added

DIRECTIONS

1. preheat oven to 350 Fahrenheit. Line the baking sheet along with some parchment paper.

2. In a medium mixing cup, add all ingredients and pound on low speed with the handheld blender until completely mixed.

3. Chill for 30 minutes in the refrigerator.

   5. Take out of the fridge & break into six equivalent parts. Make a ball out of each section and put it on the prepared baking sheet.

   6. Chill for 2 hrs in the refrigerator. Switch to the airtight jar and hold refrigerated for up to one week before ready to feed.

NUTRITION: Calories: 131 Cal Fat: 10 g Protein: 3 g Carbs: 7 g

8. Swedish Meatballs

Ready in: 30 minutes

Servings: 5

Difficulty: Easy

INGREDIENTS

Meatballs

- 1/2 cup of breadcrumbs

- One large egg

- 1/2 cup of (125ml) milk

- 35 ml cream

- 1/3 tsp salt

- 1 tbsp garlic

- 1/4 tsp black pepper & ground white pepper each

- 1/4 tsp Grillkrydda / allspice / all-purpose seasoning

- 1/2 cup of finely chopped onion

- 1 lb. ground beef

- 1/2 lb. ground pork

- 2 tbsps finely chopped fresh parsley

- 2 tsp olive oil

- 1 tbsp butter

Gravy Sauce

- 1/3 cup of butter

- 1/4 cup of plain/all-purpose flour

- 250 ml beef broth (or stock)

- 250 ml vegetable broth

- 1 cup thickened cream

- 2 tsp soy sauce

- Salt & pepper

- 1 tsp Dijon mustard

DIRECTIONS

1. Combine the breadcrumbs, peppers, garlic, milk, egg, cinnamon, cream, and seasoning in a large mixing cup. Give at least 10 minutes for the milk to sink into the breadcrumbs.

2. Substitute the carrot, meat(s), & parsley after milk has consumed some of the oil. To blend, blend very well using your fingertips.

3. Shape the meat into roughly 24 tiny or 16 bigger balls.

4. In a medium-high-heat bowl, melt 1 tbsp of butter & 2 tsp of oil. To stop stewing or simmering, cook meatballs in two-batch batches. Wrap in foil and switch to the warm tray.

5. Melt the one-third cup butter in the skillet with the juices. Whisk throughout the flour till it's fully dissolved and brown in appearance. In a wide mixing cup, combine the broth, milk, soy sauce, and Dijon mustard. Season with pepper and salt to taste and carry to a boil. To blend both of the flavors, thoroughly combine the sauce.

7. Proceed to cook until the sauce has thickened.

NUTRITION: Calories: 484 Cal Fat: 41 g Protein: 18 g Carbs: 9 g

9. Scrambled Egg Wraps

Ready in: 20 minutes

Servings: 6

Difficulty: Easy

INGREDIENTS

- One chopped sweet red pepper

- One chopped green pepper

- 2 tsp canola oil

- Five plum tomatoes, seeded & chopped

- 1/2 cup of soy milk

- 1/4 tsp salt

- Six eggs

- Six tortillas

DIRECTIONS

1. Sauté peppers into the oil until soft in a broad nonstick skillet. Cook for the next 1 to 2 minutes after inserting the tomatoes. Whisk the soy milk, eggs, and salt together in a large mixing cup. Reduce the heat to mild and pour in the egg mixture. Cook, stirring continuously until the eggs are ready. Top each tortilla with 2/3 cup of the mixture and roll them up.

NUTRITION: Calories: 258 Cal Fat: 10 g Protein: 12 g Carbs: 30 g

10. Falafel

Ready in: 50 minutes

Servings: 1

Difficulty: Medium

INGREDIENTS

- 2 cups of dried chickpeas

- ½ tsp baking soda

- 1 cup parsley

- ¾ cup cilantro

- ½ cup dill

- One quartered small onion

- 7-8 peeled garlic cloves

- Salt

- 1 tbsp ground black pepper

- 1 tbsp ground cumin

- 1 tbsp ground coriander

- optional 1 tsp cayenne pepper

- 1 tsp baking powder

- 2 tbsp toasted sesame seeds

- Oil for frying

Falafel Sauce

- Tahini Sauce

Fixings for falafel sandwich (optional)

- Pita pockets

- Chopped or diced English cucumbers

- Tomatoes, chopped/diced

- Pickles

- Baby Arugula

DIRECTIONS

1. In a wide mixing cup, add both dried chickpeas & baking soda with sufficient water to cover the chickpeas by almost 2 inches. Soak for 18 hours overnight. When the chickpeas are finished, drain them full, then pat those dry.

2. In a wide bowl of the food processor equipped with a blade, mix the garlic, onions, herbs, chickpeas, and spices. Run the food processor for 40 seconds before all of the ingredients are well mixed and the falafel mixture is created.

3. Put that falafel mixture in a bowl and securely cover. Refrigerate for almost 1 hour (or up to one night) before cooking.

4. Add sesame seeds and baking powder to a falafel mixture well before frying and whisk with a spoon.

5. Scoop falafel mixture then shapes into 12-inch-thick patties. It's simpler to shape the patties with wet hands.

6. Dump 3 inches of oil into a medium saucepan. Heat this oil over medium to high heat until it gently bursts. Drop these falafel patties into the oil carefully and fry for 3-5 minutes, or until crispy and medium brown outside. If required, fry this falafel in batches to prevent crowding the plate.

8. Drain that fried-falafel patty in the colander or on a paper towel-lined pan.

9. Organize falafel patties into pita bread with tomato, hummus or tahini, arugula, and cucumbers, or assemble falafel patties into pita bread and hummus tahini, tomato, arugula, and cucumbers.

NUTRITION: Calories: 93 Cal Fat: 3.8 g Protein: 3.9 g Carbs: 1.4 g

11. Granola Bars

Ready in: 15 minutes

Servings: 2-4

Difficulty: Easy

INGREDIENTS

- One heaping cup of packed dates

- 1 1/2 cups of rolled oats

- 1/4 cup of creamy salted natural peanut butter /almond butter

- 1/4 cup of maple syrup /agave nectar

- 1 cup of roasted unsalted almonds

- Chocolate chips, nuts, banana chips, dried fruit, vanilla, etc.

DIRECTIONS

1. Pulse dates before little pieces remain in the food processor. This should have the strength of the dough.

1. Optional second step: In a 350 Fahrenheit oven, toast the oats for 10 to 15 minutes or until golden brown. If you don't want to toast them, keep them raw.

2. In a wide mixing cup, combine the peas, almonds, and dates; set aside.

3. In a saucepan above low heat, melt the maple syrup & peanut butter. Stir & pour over the oat mixture, then stir to spread the dates equally.

4. Switch to an 8" baking dish or the other compact pan lined in parchment paper or plastic wrap so they can be quickly extracted.

5. Force down tightly until evenly flattened – then press down & stack the bars with something flat, similar to a drinking glass, which makes them stay together easier.

6. Cover with plastic wrap or parchment paper & ice or freeze for 15 to 20 minutes to firm up.

7. Detach bars from the pan and break into ten equal bars. For up to a few days, pack in the airtight jar.

NUTRITION: Calories: 231 kcal Fat: 9.7 g Protein: 5.8 g Carbs: 33.9 g

12. Eggplant Hash with eggs

Ready in: 20 minutes

Servings: 5

Difficulty: Easy

INGREDIENTS

- Black pepper to taste

- 2 tbsp olive oil

- 8 oz chopped cheese

- Salt to taste

- ½ chopped onion

- One sliced eggplant

- 4 tbsp butter

- Eight egg

- ½ tsp soy sauce

DIRECTIONS

The Execution

1. Add the olive oil & onion to the frying pan. Sauté till onion is soft.

2. Add the eggplant & halloumi cheese to the pan & cook till everything is golden brown, occasionally stirring—season with salt & pepper to taste. When finished, plate the hash & cover to keep warm.

3. Put the eggs over the eggplant hash. Serve with remaining butter from the pan & Worcestershire sauce. Season with additional salt & pepper if desired.

NUTRITION: Calories: 554 kcal Fat: 43.6 g Protein: 36.1 g Carbs: 6.0 g

13. Easy Nachos

Ready in: 25 minutes

Servings: 8

Difficulty: Easy

INGREDIENTS

- ½ cup Black olives

- One packet Tortilla Chips

- 1 cup Beef

- 1 lb cheese

- 1 cup Chopped chicken

- 1/3 cup Tomatoes chili

- ½ cup Beans

DIRECTIONS

1. Preheat oven to 350 Fahrenheit.

2. Line a baking sheet with foil.

3. Now spread chips over it.

4. Then you sprinkle 1/2 of the grated cheese over the chips.

5. Again sprinkle toppings over the chips & cheese.

6. Sprinkle now the remaining cheese.

7. Bake it for around 10 mins, or till cheese is melty good.

8. Serve it warm with sides such as sour cream or salsa.

NUTRITION: Calories: 447 kcal Fat: 26 g Protein: 17 g Carbs: 38 g

14. Homemade ketchup

Ready in: 12 hours 10 minutes

Servings: 48

Difficulty: Difficult

INGREDIENTS

- One clove

- 28 oz chopped tomatoes

- 2/3 cup sugar

- ½ cup water

- ¾ cup vinegar

- ½ tsp garlic paste

- 1 tsp onion paste

- Salt to taste

- Black pepper to taste

- 1/8 tsp mustard powder

DIRECTIONS

1. First of all, pour some ground tomatoes into a slow cooker. Swirl 1/4 cup of water in each emptied container & place it into the slow cooker. Add some sugar, celery salt, garlic powder, vinegar, onion powder, salt, black pepper, mustard powder, cayenne pepper, & whole clove; whisk to combine.

2. Cook it on high flame, uncovered, till mixture is reduced by 1/2 & very thick, 10- 12 hrs. Stir well every hr. or so.

3. Smooth this texture of ketchup using a blender, around 20 seconds.

4. Now shift the strained ketchup in a bowl. Cool it thoroughly before tasting to adjust salt, cayenne pepper/ black pepper.

NUTRITION: Calories: 16 kcal Fat: g Protein: 0.5 g Carbs: 3.9 g

15. Greek Tzatziki

Ready in: 15 minutes

Servings: 5

Difficulty: Easy

INGREDIENTS

- 1 tbsp dill

- ½ sliced cucumber

- 4 tbsp chopped garlic

- 1 ½ cup yogurt

- 2 tbsp olive oil

- Salt to taste

- 2 tbsp vinegar

DIRECTIONS

1. Firstly, grate the cucumber & drain it through a fine-mesh overnight in the fridge.

2. Now mix the yogurt, vinegar, garlic, oil, & salt in a wide bowl. Cover & refrigerate it overnight.

3. Now shifted this grated cucumber & fresh yogurt mixture & stir to combine. So now you serve it chilled with pita bread for dipping.

NUTRITION: Calories: 75 kcal Fat: 6 g Protein: 4 g Carbs: 3 g

Chapter 19: Soup Recipes

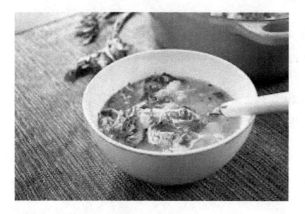

1. Beef Barley Vegetable Soup

Ready in: 360 minutes

Servings: 10

Difficulty: Easy

INGREDIENTS

- 3 lb beef

- One bay leaf

- ½ cup barley

- 2 tbsp oil

- Three diced celery stalk

- Three diced carrot

- One diced onion

- 4 cups water

- 16 oz mixed vegetables

- Black pepper as required

- Four cubes of bouillon

- 1 tbsp sugar

- 28 oz diced tomatoes

- ¼ tsp black pepper

- Salt as required

DIRECTIONS

1. For 5 hours, cook chuck roast in a slow cooker until it tender. Add bay and barley leaf in it when cooking reaches its last hour. Chop the meat into small pieces after removing it. Remove bay leaf and set the barley, beef, and broth aside.

2. On medium heat, heat oil in a wide stockpot. Cook carrots, onions, mixed vegetables, and celery until they tender. Add beef bouillon, water, sugar, pepper, chopped tomatoes, and barley mixture. Heat it until it boils, then reduce heat till it simmers for 20 minutes. To impart some more taste, use pepper and salt. Serve and enjoy the meal.

NUTRITION: Calories: 321 cal Fat: 17.3 g Protein: 20 g Carbs: 23 g

2. Hearty Vegetable Stew

Ready in: 60 minutes

Servings: 6

Difficulty: Medium

INGREDIENTS

Sauté Mixture

- Six minced garlic clove

- 3 tbsp olive oil

- Two sliced celery stalk

- One chopped onion

- Two diced carrots

Rouz mixture

- 4 cups vegetable stock

- Black pepper as required

- 1 tbsp chopped sage

- 1 tbsp chopped rosemary

- 1 tbsp chopped thyme

- ¼ cup wine

- ¼ cup rice flour

Vegetable stew

- 1 cup peas

- 2 cups chopped sweet potato

- 2 tbsp tomato paste

- Four chopped red potato

- 1 tsp marmite

- 1 tbsp soy sauce

- 1 tsp liquid smoke

- 1 tsp salt

- 1 tbsp yeast

- 2 tbsp wine

DIRECTIONS

1. Heat Olive oil in a pot over a medium flame and then add carrot, onion, and celery. Cook them until the onions are soft; it may take 9 minutes. Then add fresh herbs, garlic, and black pepper and cook again for almost 3 minutes.

2. Add flour and keep stirring to coat the added vegetables, cook for one more minute, and do not stop stirring. Now pour the white wine and add vegetable broth slowly with a quarter of a

cup at a time. It is important to keep stirring to avoid lump formation between flour and liquid.

3. Stir the tomato paste, marmite, nutritional yeast, potato, liquid smoke, soy sauce, sweet potato, boil it gently, and then simmer. Cook, it uncovered for about 30 minutes until the vegetables are tendered and keep stirring while cooking.

4. Stir the red wine vinegar and frozen peas, and then set them to cook for about 6 minutes until the peas are tender. Sprinkle some salt and pepper to impart taste to the meal. Serve the product hot and enjoy the meal.

NUTRITION: Calories: 286 cal Fat: 7 g Protein: 7 g Carbs: 48 g

3. Butternut Squash Soup

Ready in: 50 minutes

Servings: 7

Difficulty: Easy

INGREDIENTS

- ½ cup coconut milk

- 2 cups vegetable broth

- One chopped carrot

- Four minced garlic clove

- One chopped smith apple

- One chopped onion

- ¼ tsp black pepper

- 3 lb chopped butternut squash

- One sage sprig

- ¼ tsp cinnamon

- ½ tsp salt

- 1/8 tsp cayenne pepper

- ¼ tsp nutmeg

DIRECTIONS

1. Add all the ingredients to the small slow cooker and heat them for 8 hours at low flame or heat until ingredients are tender and are capable of mashing with folk at ease. Abolish the sage and stir with coconut milk.

2. With the help of an immersion blender, puree soup to the point that it becomes smooth. Taste it and add salt or pepper as desired. Serve and enjoy the meal.

NUTRITION: Calories: 305 cal Fat: 6.8 g Protein: 6.9 g Carbs: 60 g

4. Chicken Cordon Blew Soup

Ready in: 20 minutes

Servings: 8

Difficulty: Easy

INGREDIENTS

- 3 cups chicken stock

- ¼ cup butter

- One minced garlic clove

- ½ chopped onion

- ¼ cup flour

- 2 cups half and half

- 8 oz cream cheese

- 2 cup chicken, rotisserie

- One ¼ cup grated cheese, Swiss

- 1 cup chopped ham

DIRECTIONS

1. Take a large pot, melt butter in it, and then add diced onion in it. Cook until the onion gets soften. Then add garlic and heat the mixture for 1 minute, followed by flour, and put it for one more minute.

2. Draw chicken pieces into the pot slowly and add cream cheese into the pot and stir it. Stir Swiss cheese until it gets melted. Stir the ham and chicken until heated. Now serve the meal hot and enjoy it.

NUTRITION: Calories: 507 cal Fat: 26 g Protein: 34 g Carbs: 37 g

5. Swedish Meatballs with Cream of Mushroom Soup

Ready in: 35 minutes

Servings: 6

Difficulty: Easy

INGREDIENTS

Meatballs

- One egg

- ½ cup bread crumbs

- 2 tbsp olive oil

- One diced onion

- 1 tbsp diced parsley

- ½ lb lean pork

- 1 lb lean beef

- ¼ cup milk

- 1 tsp salt

- ¼ tsp nutmeg

- ½ tsp garlic powder

- 1/8 tsp allspice

- ¼ tsp black pepper

For frying

- 1 tbsp Worcestershire sauce

- 1 tbsp olive oil

- Mushroom Sauce

- 2 tbsp butter

- 1 cup beef stock

- ¼ cup sour cream

- 1 cup mushroom cream soup

DIRECTIONS

1. Take a large-sized skillet, and on medium heat, roast crumbs of bread while stirring it continuously. The toasty smell and dark brown color of bread will indicate that it has been roasted. Now transfer it to a large mixing bowl.

2. Now heat Olive oil in the skillet and add and cook onions in it for three minutes. Sprinkle a salt pinch and pepper to impart taste and move it to the bowl of breadcrumbs.

3. Now add milk, parsley, ground meat, egg, spices, and salt to the onion and bread crumb mixture. Mesh the mixture well.

4. Convert the meat mixture in the form of meatballs of some even size. Place them on a plate and set them aside.

5. On medium heat, melt butter and oil in a skillet. Now cook the meatballs in till they turn brown.

6. Now to clean the skillet, pour the broth and bring it to a boil so that stirring could help remove these scraps from the bottom of the skillet. If you are using a non-stick pan, it won't be an issue then.

7. Now stir the sour and mushroom cream.

8. Then put back the meatball into the pan and mitigate the heat and cook it for 6 minutes.

9. Your meatballs are ready now and serve them while they are hot. Serve them with noodles, and never forget to pour sauce and sprinkle parsley over it. Serve and enjoy the meal.

NUTRITION: Calories: 409 kcal Fat: 10 g Protein: 27 g Carbs: 12 g

6. Swedish Meatballs Soup

Ready in: 50 minutes

Servings: 6

Difficulty: Easy

INGREDIENTS

Meatballs

- ¼ cup diced parsley

- 1 lb beef

- ½ cup ricotta cheese

- 1 lb ground turkey

- Two eggs

- 1 tsp salt

- ½ cup breadcrumbs

- ½ tsp pepper

- ¼ tsp nutmeg

- ¼ tsp allspice

Soup

- 8 oz pasta

- One sliced onion

- 1/3 cup flour

- 6 tbsp butter

- ½ tsp nutmeg

- 6 cups beef broth

- ½ tsp allspice

- ½ cup heavy cream

- Salt to taste

- 1 cup sour cream

- Black pepper to taste

- 2 tbsp diced parsley

- Dill weed as required

DIRECTIONS

1. Heat oven up to 400 Fahrenheit.

2. Now mix the ingredients of the meatball in a bowl.

3. Form the mixture into the size of walnut balls and put the meatballs into the baking dish. Bake them for 25 minutes until they are cooked.

4. Cook onion in melted butter in a Dutch Oven of large size until they are tender. Then remove them from the pot.

5. Stir Spices, flour, and the nutmeg in the butter remained behind and cooked for 2 minutes.

6. Pour broth and cook it while stirring until it gets thickened. Add meatballs and bring them to a simmer.

7. Now follow the instructions on package cook pasta.

8. Along with heavy sour cream and parsley, stir the pasta into the pot. Season the meat with pepper and salt according to your taste.

9. Fill the bowl with soup and serve it hot and enjoy it.

NUTRITION: Calories: 656 cal Fat: 31.5 g Protein: 30 g Carbs: 60.5 g

7. Potato Cauliflower and Ham Soup

Ready in: 35 minutes

Servings: 5

Difficulty: Easy

INGREDIENTS

- 1 cup grated cheese

- 5 ½ cups diced cauliflower

- 2 cups diced broccoli

- 5 cups chopped russet potatoes

- 1 tsp salt

- 1/3 cup chopped celery

- 8 cups water

- 5 cups chopped ham, cooked

- 6 tbsp flour

- 4 tbsp chicken bouillon

- 6 tbsp butter

- 2 ½ cups milk

- 2 tsp black pepper

DIRECTIONS

1. Mix all the ingredients in a stockpot. Boil the ingredients and then cover the pot and mitigate the heat level. Boil them for 12 minutes until they are soft. Stir it in the pepper, chicken bouillon, and salt. With the help of a fork, break cauliflower and potatoes into small pieces.

2. Melt the butter in a separate saucepan at medium heat. Add Sweep flour in it and cook for 2 minutes until the mixture gets thick. Now stir it in the cheese and milk for 6 minutes.

3. Stir the mixture of milk in the stockpot and then cook the soup.

4. Then garnish it with cheddar cheese.

NUTRITION: Calories: 257 cal Fat: 10 g Protein: 21 g Carbs: 6 g

8. Chicken Tortilla Soup

Ready in: 40 minutes

Servings: 8

Difficulty: Easy

INGREDIENTS

- 1 cup corn

- 1 tbsp olive oil

- Three minced garlic clove

- One diced onion

- One chopped jalapeno

- 1 tsp chili powder

- 1 tsp cumin

- 14 ½ oz mashed tomatoes

- 3 cup chicken stock

- 2 tbsp lime juice

- 2 cups chopped tomatoes

- 14 ½ oz black beans

- 2 lb chicken boneless pieces

- ¼ cup diced cilantro

- One diced avocado

DIRECTIONS

1. Heat Olive oil at medium heat in a pan. Add and fry tortilla strips in stages until they are crisp, and then drain it and sprinkle with a salt pinch.

2. Now at medium flame, heat olive oil, add jalapeno, onion, and garlic, and cook them until they get soft.

3. Add all the ingredients which remained behind and let it simmer for 25 minutes, or the chicken is cooked.

4. Remove and shred the chicken, and then add it back into the stockpot and let it simmer for 4 minutes.

5. Pour the soup into the bowl and mix it with sliced avocado, tortilla strips, and lime wedges.

NUTRITION: Calories: 278 cal Fat: 11 g Protein: 18 g Carbs: 27 g

9. Mulligatawny Soup

Ready in: 80 minutes

Servings: 6

Difficulty: Medium

INGREDIENTS

- ½ cup heavy cream

- ½ cup diced onion

- One chopped carrot

- Two diced celery stalks

- ¼ cup butter

- 1 ½ tsp curry powder

- 1 ½ tbsp all-purpose flour

- 4 cups chicken stock

- ¼ cup rice

- ½ chopped apple

- 2 lb chicken boneless pieces

- Salt to taste

- ¼ tsp thyme, dried

- Black pepper to taste

DIRECTIONS

1. Cook onions, carrot, butter, and celery in the pot of soup. Then add curry and flour and then cook it for 6 minutes. Further, add in chicken stock and boil and let it simmer for half an hour.

2. Now add rice, salt, thyme, rice, and salt, and then let it get cooked for 20 minutes.

3. Add hot cream and then serve it hot and enjoy.

NUTRITION: Calories: 223 cal Fat: 15.8 g Protein: 7 g Carbs: 13.5 g

10. Egg and Lemon Soup

Ready in: 90 minutes

Servings: 6

Difficulty: Difficult

INGREDIENTS

- ¼ cup Lemon juice

- 1 kg Chicken

- One chopped onion

- Black pepper to taste

- 8 cup water

- ½ cup chopped orzo

- Salt to taste

- Four egg

For Serving

- Black pepper

- Oregano

- ½ lemon

DIRECTIONS

1. Bake chicken, and it is stock with peppercorns chicken, salt, water, and onion, and baked chicken for 60 minutes. Then strain the chicken broth, and shred them into pieces to the chicken. Now bake orzo in the broth for 9 to 20 minutes; after that, made the avgolemono by placing the egg in lemon juice and add into the soup. Then mix the avgolemono into chicken orzo and stir to combine it, thicken it for 3 to minutes, and don't boil. Serve it with a lemon slice, oregano, and black pepper.

NUTRITION: Calories: 431 kcal Fat: 28.2 g Protein: 30.7 g Carbs: 12.8 g

11. Seafood Bisque

Ready in: 30 minutes

Servings: 10

Difficulty: Easy

INGREDIENTS

- Onion to chopped

- Two can Mushroom soup

- 3 tbsp chicken soup

- Two cups of celery soup

- 6 oz crabmeat

- 2 2/3 cup milk

- Four crushed onion

- 11/2 lb chopped shrimp

- ½ crushed celery

Pepper to taste

- One clove chopped Garlic

- ¼ tsp chili sauce

- 1 tsp sauce

DIRECTIONS

1. mix all eight components, boil them, combine shrimp, mushrooms, and carbs and boil it for 9 to 20 minutes. Mix them in wine, salt, and pepper and cook for 2 to 3 minutes. Serve online and enjoy.

NUTRITION: Calories: 169 kcal Fat: 6 g Protein: 18 g Carbs: 10 g

12. Sausage Potato and Kale Soup

Ready in: 60 minutes

Servings: 12

Difficulty: Medium

INGREDIENTS

- 1 lb Italian sausage

- 2 cups kale leaves

- 4 cups cream (half and a half)

- ½ tsp black pepper

- ½ tsp red Chili

- 3 cups chopped tomatoes

- ½ tsp chopped Oregano

- 2 cups chicken soup

- One crushed onion

- 2 cups milk

DIRECTIONS

1. In a pot, add crumble sausage and cook it for 8 minutes. Combine red pepper flakes, potatoes, oregano, chicken broth, onion, and milk and boil them for half an hour. Serve with black pepper after boiling for 15 minutes.

NUTRITION: Calories: 266 kcal Fat: 18 g Protein: 10.6 g Carbs: 16.4 g

13. Seafood Cioppino

Ready in: 165 minutes

Servings: 8

Difficulty: Difficult

INGREDIENTS

- 1 lb Cod Fillets

- ¼ cup olive oil

- 10 oz scallops

- One crushed onion

- 25 shrimp

- Four cloves chopped garlic

- 25 mussels, drained

- One crushed bell pepper

- 10 oz clam juice

- 1 cup wine

- One green chili

- ½ crushed Parsley

- 1 tsp cayenne Pepper

- Salt to taste

- 1 tsp Paprika

- Black pepper to taste

- 2 tsp chopped basil

- ½ cup water

- 1 tsp chopped oregano

- 1 tsp thyme

- One can of tomato sauce

- Two cups of chopped tomatoes

DIRECTIONS

1. In a pan cook oil, with pepper, onion, bell pepper, and garlic; mix the juice of calm, parsley, cayenne pepper, salt, paprika, pepper, water, basil, tomato sauce, oregano, thyme, and tomatoes, and boil for 60 to 120 minutes. Finally, combine scallops, clams, cod, prawns, and mussels and mix serve and enjoy it.

NUTRITION: Calories: 303 kcal Fat: 9.1 g Protein: 34.3 g Carbs: 16.5 g

14. Turkey chili Taco Soup

Ready in: 20 minutes

Servings: 9

Difficulty: Easy

INGREDIENTS

- 2 ½ chicken soup

- 1.3 lb grounded Turkey

- One packet taco seasoning

- 16 oz beans

- One crushed Onion

- One crushed bell pepper

- 8 oz tomato sauce

- 10 oz tomatoes chili

- 15 oz Kidney Beans

- 15 oz chopped frozen corn

DIRECTIONS

1. in a pan, cook onion in oil for 4 minutes, mix taco seasoning tomatoes, bean, corn, and chicken broth, and boil them for 16 to 20 minutes. Serve the soup with topping like fat sour cream, cheese, onions.

NUTRITION: Calories: 225 kcal Fat: 2 g Protein: 22 g Carbs: 31.5 g

Chapter 20: Salad Recipes

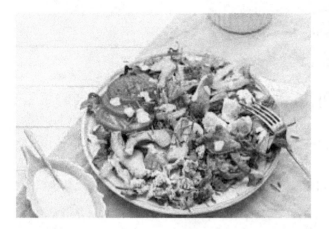

1. Green beans and Heart of Palm

Ready in 20 minutes

Servings: 8

Difficulty: Easy

INGREDIENTS

- ½ cup of chopped basil

- 1 lb. green beans

- 1 cup olives

- 1-1/2 cups of sliced palms

- ¾ crumbled cheese

- One lemon juice

- ½ cup of chopped oregano

- 1tbsp vinegar

- 1/3 cup of olive oil

DIRECTIONS

1. Boil green beans in salted water for 3-4 minutes. Drain and keep aside to cool.

2. Mix the vinegar, olive oil, oregano, basil, and lemon juice to make the dressing.

3. Take a large bowl and mix all the ingredients.

4. Toss well.

5. Serve and enjoy.

NUTRITION: Calories: 40 cal Fat: 3 g Protein: 4 g Carbs: 5 g

2. Crab Pasta

Ready in: 10 minutes

Servings: 4

Difficulty: Easy

INGREDIENTS

- 3 tbsp of olive oil

- 225g pasta

- Handful of parsley

- Red pepper flakes

- 225g crabmeat

- One garlic clove

DIRECTIONS

1. Boil pasta according to the given instructions. Drain and keep aside.

2. Chop parsley leaves.

3. Cook garlic in 2-3 tbsp olive oil in a saucepan.

4. At low heat, add pasta, crab meat, and all other ingredients and cook till all the ingredients are well mixed and softened.

5. Season with red pepper flakes.

6. Serve and enjoy.

NUTRITION: Calories: 311 cal Fat: 21 g Protein: 22 g Carbs: 6 g

3. Eggplant Salad

Ready in: 25 minutes

Servings: 2

Difficulty: Easy

INGREDIENTS

- Two garlic cloves

- Two sized eggplant

- 1-1/2 tsp salt and pepper

- One diced tomato

- 1-1/2 tsp red wine vinegar

- 3 tbsp olive oil

- ½ tsp chopped oregano

- Pita bread to serve

- Capers

DIRECTIONS

1. Take a grill and heat over medium flame. Place eggplant and prick with a fork and cook for 10-15 minutes till the skin is blistered.

2. Scoop out the eggplant.

3. Take a large bowl and mix all the ingredients.

4. Season with salt and pepper.

5. Use capers to garnish.

6. Serve with bread.

7. Enjoy.

NUTRITION: Calories: 156 cal Fat: 95 g Protein: 1.8 g Carbs: 16 g

4. Creamy Cucumber Salad

Ready in: 10 minutes

Servings: 8

Difficulty: Easy

INGREDIENTS

- ½ tsp of sugar

- 2-3 cucumbers

- ½ cup of sour cream

- 1/3 sliced onions

- ¼ cup chopped dill

- Salt to taste

- 3 tbsp white vinegar

DIRECTIONS

1. Peel and cut the cucumbers.

2. Take a large bowl and combine all the ingredients.

3. Toss well and refrigerate for 50-60 minutes.

4. Serve and enjoy.

NUTRITION: Calories: 77 cal Fat: 7 g Protein: 1 g Carbs: 4 g

5. Spinach with Egg and Bacon

Ready in: 10 minutes

Servings: 6

Difficulty: Easy

INGREDIENTS

- Six eggs

- 480 g cherry tomatoes

- 1tbsp olive oil

- 250g bacon

- 240g spinach

- Six toasted bread slices

- 1tbsp white vinegar

DIRECTIONS

1. Take a baking dish.

2. Put baking paper sprayed with oil and palace tomatoes in it.

3. Bake them in preheated oven for 20-25 minutes.

4. Take a pan and cook bacon for 2-3 minutes.

5. Transfer it to the plate.

6. Now cook spinach with 1 tbsp of olive oil in the pan for 2-3 minutes.

7. Boil water, adds a spoon of vinegar and carefully crack the egg in a separate small bowl and drop in the pan's middle.

8. Cook all the eggs and transfer them to the six serving plates.

9. Top with remaining ingredients.

10. Season with salt and black pepper.

11. Serve and enjoy.

NUTRITION: Calories: 55 Cal Fat: 15 g Protein: 21 g Carbs: 4 g

6. Buffalo Chicken Salad

Ready in: 60 minutes

Servings: 4

Difficulty: moderate

INGREDIENTS

Meat ingredients

- 2tbsp honey

- 1cup buffalo sauce

- Salt

- 1tbsp olive oil

- 1 lb. boneless chicken

- Black pepper

- ½ tsp onion powder

- One lime juice

- 1 tsp garlic powder

Dressing ingredients

- ½ tsp. black pepper

- ½ cup mayonnaise

- 1/2 cup buttermilk

- ½ cream

- ¼ cup chopped parsley

- Two minced garlic cloves

- ½ tbsp salt

- 2 tbsp chopped chives

- Cayenne pepper

Salad ingredients

- ¼ cup crumbled cheese

- 4 cup chopped romaine

- Two sliced celery

- 2 cup spinach

- One carrot

- ½ sliced onion

- One cucumber

- 1 cup cherry tomatoes

DIRECTIONS

1. Take a large bowl and mix meat, honey, lemon juice, onion, and garlic powder. Add salt and pepper to taste.

2. Add chicken meat to marinade.

3. Toss well.

4. Keep aside for 25-30 minutes at room temperature.

5. Heat oil in a skillet over medium flame and cook chicken for 10-20 minutes.

6. Place the cooked chicken on a chopping board and make small pieces of it.

7. Take a bowl and mix mayonnaise, cream & buttermilk. Put other ingredients and stir well.

8. Keep in the refrigerator for 50 minutes.

9. Mix all the salad ingredients in a large bowl.

10. Top the salad with cooked chicken and serve.

11. Enjoy.

NUTRITION: Calories: 291 cal Fat: 10.8 g Protein: 31.6g Carbs: 15 g

7. Cobb Egg Salad

Ready in: 20 minutes

Servings: 6

Difficulty: Easy

INGREDIENTS

- Eight crumbled bacon strips

- 3 tbsp. mayonnaise

- 3tbsp. yogurt

- Salt to taste

- 2-3 tbsp red wine vinegar

- Eight boiled eggs

- pepper to taste

- One sliced avocado

- ½ cherry tomatoes

- ½ crumbled cheese

- 2 tbsp chopped chives

DIRECTIONS

1. Take a bowl and mix mayonnaise, vinegar, and yogurt.

2. Sprinkle salt and pepper.

3. Mix the remaining ingredients in a large bowl.

4. Add mayonnaise mixture.

5. Mix well.

6. Garnish with chopped chives.

7. Serve and enjoy.

NUTRITION: Calories: 235 cal Fat: 16.7 g Protein: 13.5 g Carbs: 8.8 g

8. Chinese Chicken Salad

Ready in: 15 minutes

Servings: 3

Difficulty: Easy

INGREDIENTS

Dressing ingredients

- 2 tbsp soy sauce

- 1tbsp toasted sesame oil

- 3 tbsp of rice vinegar

- One garlic clove

- 2 tbsp of grapeseed oil

- 1-1/2 tsp minced ginger

- 1 tsp of sugar

- ½ tsp of pepper

Salad ingredients

- 1 cup of carrot

- 4 cups of cabbage

- Two cups of chicken

- 1-1/2 cups of red cabbage

- ½ cups of shallots

Garnishes

- 2-3 tsp of sesame seeds

- ½ cup of crunchy noodles

DIRECTIONS

1. Take a jar and gently mix the dressing ingredients and keep aside for 10-15 minutes.

2. Take a large bowl and mix the salad ingredients with crunchy noodles.

3. Drizzle with dressing.

4. Toss well.

5. Distribute in the serving bowls and garnish with crunchier noodles.

6. Serve and enjoy.

NUTRITION: Calories: 412 cal Fat: 23.2 g Protein: 32.3 g Carbs: 17.3 g

9. Loaded Italian Salad

Ready in: 20 minutes

Servings: 3

Difficulty: Easy

INGREDIENTS

- ¼ cup of water

- One pack Italian mix dressing

- Half tsp sugar

- ½ tsp Italian dried seasoning

- 1/3 tsp garlic powder

- 1/3 cup of white vinegar

- ¾ cup of vegetable oil

- ½ tsp salt

- pepper

- ½ tbsp of mayonnaise

DIRECTIONS

1. Take a bowl and mix all the ingredients.

2. Shake well to combine.

3. Serve and enjoy.

NUTRITION: Calories: 630 cal Fat: 35 g Protein: 29 g Carbs: 49 g

10. Dill Cucumber Salad

Ready in: 1:00-15 minutes

Servings: 8

Difficulty: Easy

INGREDIENTS

- 2 tsp red wine vinegar

- One lb cucumbers

- 2 tsp salt

- ½ peeled red onions

- 2 tsp sugar

- 2 tsp balsamic vinegar

- ½ cup of water

- 2 tsp apple cider vinegar

- ¼ cup of chopped dill leaves

DIRECTIONS

1. Take a bowl and mix sliced cucumbers, salt, sugar, and pepper. Place in the fridge for 60 minutes.

2. Take out from the refrigerator and drain.

3. Add other ingredients and mix.

4. Serve and enjoy.

NUTRITION: Calories: 16 cal Fat: 1 g Protein: 1 g Carbs: 3 g

11. Cucumber Avocado Salad with Lime Mint and Feta

Ready in: 35 minutes

Servings: 4

Difficulty: Easy

INGREDIENTS

- 2-3 chopped avocados

- 2 cups of chopped cucumbers

- ½ cup of chopped mint

- Pinch of salt

- One lime juice

- ½ cup of crumbled feta

For dressing

- 1 tbsp lime juice

- 2 tbsp olive oil

DIRECTIONS

1. Cut the cucumbers.

2. Season with salt and pepper. Keep aside for 30-35 minutes.

3. Drain them and add olive oil and lime juice.

4. Mix well.

5. Mix all the ingredients in a large bowl.

6. Add dressing and mix well.

7. Serve and enjoy.

NUTRITION: Calories: 289 cal Fat: 26 g Protein: 5 g Carbs: 14 g

12. Avocado Egg Salad

Ready in: 25 minutes

Servings: 2

Difficulty: Easy

INGREDIENTS

- Lettuce leaves

- One diced avocado

- 2tbsp chopped red onion

- Three boiled eggs

- 1 tbsp chopped chives

- 2tbsp mayonnaise

- Salt

- 1 tbsp chopped parsley

- 1tsp lemon juice

- pepper to taste

DIRECTIONS

1. Take a large bowl and mix all the ingredients.

2. Serve with bread topped with lettuce leaves.

3. Enjoy.

NUTRITION: Calories: 119 cal Fat: 8.7 g Protein: 7.2 g Carbs: 3.4 g

13. Red Cabbage and Egg Salad

Ready in: 30 minutes

Servings: 3

Difficulty: Easy

INGREDIENTS

- ½ tsp salt

- Five diced carrots

- ½ red cabbage

- Four boiled eggs

- One red pepper-small

- ½ chopped parsley

- One chopped red onion

- pepper

For dressing

- 1 tsp ground sugar

- 2 tbsp of mayonnaise

- 3-4 tbsp yogurt

- 1 tbsp apple cider vinegar

- 1-2 tbsp salad cream

DIRECTIONS

1. Cut the cabbage.

2. Take a large mixing bowl and mix diced boiled eggs, cabbage, dressing, and other remaining ingredients.

3. Add parsley.

4. Mix well.

5. Serve and enjoy.

NUTRITION: Calories: 199 cal Fat: 8.9 g Protein: 14.6 g Carbs: 19.9 g

14. Strawberry Jello

Ready in: 40 minutes

Servings: 10

Difficulty: Easy

INGREDIENTS

- Nine oz. mix strawberry jello

- Eight oz. cooled whip

- One lb. strawberries

DIRECTIONS

1. Take mix jello powder and one cup of boiling water in a large mixing bowl followed by 1-cup cold water.

2. Stir well till the jello is melted.

3. Place it in the refrigerator.

4. Let the mixture set well.

5. Add cooled whip and stir so that everything combines well.

6. Take a springform pan and spray it with oil. Add the mixture in it and place halved strawberries on the top.

7. Refrigerate for 30 minutes.

8. Mix 1-cup of boiled water and 3oz. Strawberry jello in a separate jar.

9. Refrigerate.

10. Put the jello mixture on the top and allow it to set.

11. Serve and enjoy.

NUTRITION: Calories: 121 cal Fat: 1 g Protein: 2 g Carbs: 27 g

15. Mac Cheeseburger Salad

Ready in: 20 minutes. minutes

Servings: 4

Difficulty: Easy

INGREDIENTS

- 1 cup cheddar

- 1 lb ground beef

- 1 tbsp of Worcestershire sauce

- Salt and ground pepper

- 1 tbsp red wine vinegar

- 1 tsp of garlic powder

- ½ cup yogurt

- One sliced tomato

- 1 tsp ketchup

- 2 tsp mustard

- ½ tsp paprika

- Two chopped lettuce

- 1 tsp sesame seeds

- ¼ sliced onion

- Quartered dill pickle

DIRECTIONS

1. Take a skillet and heat over medium flame. Add beef, sauce, salt, garlic powder, and pepper. Cook for 5-10 minutes.

2. For the dressing, mix yogurt, mustard, vinegar, paprika, and ketchup in a large bowl.

3. Assembly: mix tomatoes, romaine, pickles, onions, and cheddar in a large mixing bowl. Add dressing.

4. Use sesame seeds for garnishing.

5. Serve and enjoy.

NUTRITION: Calories: 368 cal Fat: 31 g Protein: 18 g Carbs: 3 g

Chapter 21: Smoothies Recipes

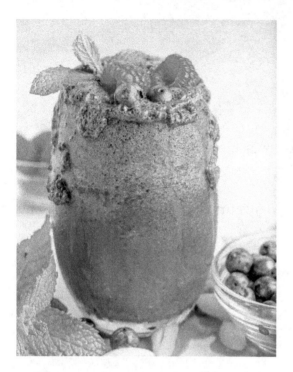

1. Frappe

Ready in: 5 minutes

Servings: 1

Difficulty: Easy

INGREDIENTS

- Ice cubes as required

- 1 ½ cup chilled coffee

- 2 tbsp sugar syrup

- ½ cup milk

- Whipped cream for serving as required

DIRECTIONS

1. Add all the ingredients to a food processor and blend to get a smooth, creamy mixture.

2. Serve with ice cream and enjoy it.

NUTRITION: Calories: 89 kcal Fat: 2 g Protein: 2 g Carbs: 16 g

2. White Wine Spritzer

Ready in: 5 minutes

Servings: 1

Difficulty: Easy

INGREDIENTS

- Lime slices for garnishing

- ¼ cup soda, chilled

- ¾ cup white wine, chilled

DIRECTIONS

1. Add wine and soda to a wine glass and stir well.

2. Serve and enjoy it.

NUTRITION: Calories: 90 cal Fat: 0 g Protein: 0 g Carbs: 3 g

3. Paloma

Ready in: 5 minutes

Servings: 1

Difficulty: Easy

INGREDIENTS

- ¼ oz sugar syrup

- 2 oz tequila

- 2 oz water, sparkling

- 2 oz grapefruit juice

- 4 tbsp lime juice

- Ice cubes as required

- Salt to taste

DIRECTIONS

1. Add all the ingredients to a food processor and blend to get a smooth mixture.

2. Serve and enjoy it.

NUTRITION: Calories: 212 cal Fat: 0 g Protein: 0 g Carbs: 17 g

4. Cherry Lime Slush

Ready in: 5 minutes

Servings: 2

Difficulty: Easy

INGREDIENTS

- ½ cup sugar

- 4 cups cherries, sweet

- 2 cups sparkling water

- ½ cup lime juice

DIRECTIONS

1. Add all the ingredients to a food processor and blend to get a smooth mixture.

2. Serve and enjoy it.

NUTRITION: Calories: 189 kcal Fat: 1 g Protein: 3 g Carbs: 49 g

5. Caipirinha Cocktail

Ready in: 5 minutes

Servings: 1

Difficulty: Easy

INGREDIENTS

- 1 tbsp lime juice

- 1 ½ sliced lime

- 2 oz cachaça

- 2 tbsp sugar

- Crushed ice

DIRECTIONS

1. Add all the ingredients to a food processor and blend to get a smooth mixture.

2. Serve and enjoy it.

NUTRITION: Calories: 196 kcal Fat: 0.5 g Protein: 0.7 g Carbs: 11.2 g

6. Ginger Peach Vodka Mule

Ready in: 5 minutes

Servings: 2

Difficulty: Easy

INGREDIENTS

- 1 cup seltzer water

- 1 tsp ginger paste

- 2 oz peach syrup

- 2 oz vodka

DIRECTIONS

1. Add all the ingredients to a food processor and blend to get a smooth mixture.

2. Serve and enjoy it.

NUTRITION: Calories: 216 cal Fat: 1 g Protein: 0 g Carbs: 31 g

7. **Starbucks Pink Drink**

Ready in: 5 minutes

Servings: 4

Difficulty: Easy

INGREDIENTS

- Strawberry slices

- 1 cup tea, herbal

- ½ cup grape juice

- 1 cup boiling water

- 1 ½ cup coconut milk

DIRECTIONS

1. Add tea bags in cups and pour in boiling water. Remove the tea bags.

2. Add grape juice, ice, and coconut milk.

3. Place strawberry slices and serve.

NUTRITION: Calories: 124 cal Fat: 5 g Protein: 2 g Carbs: 21 g

8. Honeysuckle Iced Tea

Ready in: 15 minutes

Servings: 2

Difficulty: Easy

INGREDIENTS

- Honey as required

- Two ¼ cups honeysuckle flower

- 2 cups water

- Mint as required for garnishing

DIRECTIONS

1. Boil water in the pan and turn off the flame.

2. Add flowers in boiling water and stir.

3. Cover the pan and leave it for two hours.

4. Strain the flower-soaked water and discard the debris.

5. The honeysuckle is ready.

6. You can store it in an airtight container in the fridge.

7. Add honeysuckle in glass and add in ice.

8. Stir and serve.

NUTRITION: Calories: 69 cal Fat: 0 g Protein: 0 g Carbs: 9 g

9. Chocolate Caramel Delight Smoothie

Ready in: 10 minutes

Servings: 1

Difficulty: Easy

INGREDIENTS

- 2 tbsp grated toasted coconut

- 1 cup almond milk

- 1/3 cup chocolate shake

- 1 cup crushed ice

- 1 tsp caramel extract

DIRECTIONS

1. Add all the ingredients to a food processor and blend to get a smooth mixture.

2. Serve and enjoy it.

NUTRITION: Calories: 281 cal Fat: 12 g Protein: 19 g Carbs: 22 g

Conclusion

A ketogenic diet reduces or excludes carbohydrates completely. Some carbs, on the other hand, have health benefits. People should eat a diet that contains various food items with various nutrients such as carbs, fats, proteins, minerals, vitamins, salt, and much more, which can be obtained from fruits, veggies, dairy items, and most importantly the water, for a less restrictive dietary plan.

When following a ketogenic diet, everybody must keep their protein consumption down while increasing their fat intake. As you shift to a low-carb diet, the body enters a ketosis stage, where fat instead of carbohydrates is used for energy because they breakdown slowly by the digestive system, which in turn delays the decomposition of carbs, maintain the blood glucose levels in the body, and allowing us to remain fuller much longer. According to some proof, adding a tablespoon of coconut oil to your daily diet can help you lose weight. You will also need to keep an eye on portion sizes, but since fat is naturally enticing, serving one for breakfast may help you stop overeating at other times of the day.

Eating high-fat foods, such as keto fat bombs, will help you lose weight by suppressing your hunger for the next meal. They are a dieter's wish come true, whether it's fat bombs, cheesy waffles, or some other high-fat, low-carb food. The ketogenic diet has been shown to improve brain function. Ketogenic food recipes are easy to make, preserve, and consume, and they also need fewer ingredients than some other foods. Ketogenic desserts are delicious and come with a wide range of low-carb recipes. Ketogenic recipes easy to transport and ready to eat anytime you want.

You'll find the best and easiest keto and delicious high-fat recipes in this book, which will satisfy your dessert cravings after meals or when you are not too hungry. Enjoy these recipes yourself, or better yet, share them with your friends and family.

CPSIA information can be obtained
at www.ICGtesting.com
Printed in the USA
BVHW092031030521
606332BV00007B/1489